The Ultimate Guide
To Conquering Pain

By Robert Kroening

The Ultimate Guide to Conquering Pain

By Robert Kroening

Published by Natural Health Insiders
A Division of Online Publishing & Marketing, LLC

IMPORTANT CAUTION:

By reading this special report you are demonstrating an interest in maintaining good and vigorous health.

This report suggests ways you can do that, but – as with anything in medicine – there are no guarantees.

You must check with private, professional medical advisors to assess whether the suggestions in this report are appropriate for you. And please note, the contents of this report may be considered controversial by the medical community at large.

The author, editors and publishers of this report are not doctors or professional health caregivers. They have relied on information from people who are. The information in this report is not meant to replace the attention or advice of physicians or other healthcare professionals. Nothing contained in this report is meant to constitute personal medical advice for any particular individual.

No alternative OR mainstream pain treatment can boast a one hundred percent record of success. There is ALWAYS some risk involved in any pain treatment. The author, editors, and publishers of this report are not responsible for any adverse effects or results from the use of any of the suggestions, preparations or procedures described in this report.

As with any medical treatment, results of the treatments described in this report will vary from one person to another.

PLEASE DO NOT USE THE INFORMATION FROM THIS REPORT IF YOU ARE NOT WILLING TO ASSUME THE RISK.

The author reports here the results of a vast array of treatments and research as well as the personal experiences of individual patients, healthcare professionals, and caregivers. In most cases the author was not present himself to witness the events described but relied in good faith on the accounts of the people who were.

This report is not geared to treatment of catastrophic injury or disease. Though many of the treatments described have been used to treat serious injuries, disease, and pain, their results are not identical for all patients and neither this report nor the therapies it describes are represented as all-encompassing or universally applicable.

ISBN: 978-1-4951-1004-7

ABOUT THE AUTHOR

Robert Kroening attended the U.S. Military Academy at West Point, studying civil engineering. He subsequently became an airborne ranger and senior Army aviator, flying Cobra gunships and aeroscout aircraft, and commanding the rigorous aeroscout night flight training program at Ft. Rucker, Alabama. After leaving the military, he followed the path blazed by his great-grandfather into publishing and medicine. That great-grandfather, after being blinded in a silver mining accident above Leadville, Colorado, started or owned and operated three newspapers, built three houses, and ultimately became an accomplished and well-respected osteopathic physician. His daughter also became a doctor of osteopathy, and delivered Robert in a small rural hospital she started and ran in western Colorado. Robert has been a writer, managing editor, and publisher for some of the largest and most far-reaching consumer medical newsletters in America, including *Dr. William Campbell Douglass' Second Opinion*, *Dr. David Williams' Alternatives*, *Dr. Julian Whitaker's Health and Healing*, *Dr. Stephen Sinatra's Heart, Health and Nutrition*, and *Dr. Marcus Laux's Naturally Well Today*. He presently continues his research into the latest, along with the most time-proven, medical procedures and therapies.

Contents

It's a World of Pain

Chapter 1

What We're Dealing With

There is scarcely a more universal topic than pain. We've all felt it. Many of us feel it now – some intensely. All lives are shaped by it; many lives are limited by it; some lives are effectively destroyed by it. In this report, we'll give you a number of highly effective ways to deal with it.

I won't insult you with the dictionary definition of pain. If you've felt it, you know what it is – and almost everyone has felt it. And when I say "almost," the exceptions prove the rule. Those who have nerve disorders that keep them from feeling pain know it's not a good thing. Their lives are dangerous precisely because their nerves can't tell them when they're doing themselves harm.

And that's a key point. Within that observation lies a simple truth that should always be kept in mind: *Pain is not inherently a bad thing.* Without it, we'd be in big trouble. But sometimes, like fire, it becomes too intense, lasts too long, or spreads too far. That's when it becomes a problem. That's when we need help making it go away – or at least become less severe.

An old anecdote contains a useful nugget as we consider the treatment of pain. When a patient visits his doctor, he says, "Doc, it hurts when I do this." "Well," replies the doctor, *"don't do that!"*

That's what your nerves often tell you. When they alert you that it hurts to do a given thing, they're saying, "Don't do that!" And if you want to get better, you should listen – if at all possible. It's *not* always possible, which is one of the reasons this report is necessary. But avoiding things that cause the problem is the first step to getting back to normal, and it's a *very* important first step.

Because so many types of pain are being addressed in this report, a broad spectrum of treatments will be presented. Many of these will entail visiting a health professional. If you're like me, you like do-it-yourself treatments best, and there will be many of those. But there are some excellent treatments available that require the services of a health professional. In the interest of thoroughness, and even more in the interest of relieving your pain, I will present a number of such treatments. If you don't like the idea of visiting or don't want to pay a health professional, there's still plenty here to work with.

You Already Have the Most Effective Tool for Treating Pain

By far the most important aspect of pain treatment is *the mental component*. This is not to say that pain is "all in your head." Far from it. Nor is it to say that your mind has magical powers to heal. It doesn't. It's not even to say that, if you really put your mind to it, you can put your pain behind you. In some cases, that's impossible.

The truth of the matter is much more important: You can use your mind to learn about yourself, the makeup and complexity of your body, your injury or disease, how to treat your source of pain, how to work around it while it's healing or if it doesn't heal, and how to be productive and a source of benefit to others regardless of how things go with you.

These are enormously significant accomplishments. In many cases, they will result in healing. In the remainder of cases, they will cause people to become better individuals than they were before their pain episodes. That sounds like a cop-out. It's anything but. It's a very solemn, priceless truth for those who can accept it. Don't underestimate these realms of human activity. If you can't heal your pain (and even if you can), they are what will make your life grow and deepen.

On every level, your brain is an enormously influential organ. It is the seat of your emotions and your thought processes, it controls both the automatic and voluntary actions of your body, and it's also where all the pain in your body eventually registers. This co-location of such vital and related processes makes possible some powerful steps to take in dealing with pain.

Our nerves contain millions of neurons that enable our physical sense of feeling, but the brain is estimated to contain 100 *billion* of them. A lot goes on there. Thinking, sensing, analyzing, remembering, emoting, and reasoning all occur in the brain.

Even the very conventional Mayo Pain Clinic recognizes the brain's ability to deal with pain. Retraining the mind's processes is a central element of Mayo's protocol. Patients are encouraged to stop or reduce their pain medications (which often results in a lessening of pain, ironically). They're also told to stop using "crutch" behaviors, such as (with back pain, for example) sitting down, voicing the fact that they are experiencing pain, or rubbing the area where the pain is being experienced. In short, the clinic trains people to stop making unnecessary concessions to the pain they're experiencing. This is harder than it sounds, and it doesn't sound easy. It does not always make the pain go away, but, for people who have severe, chronic pain, this is often the only thing that makes their pain bearable. It is a testament to discipline, learning, and the power of one's determination that it can be so effective.

But the biggest single way your mind can help you deal with your pain is if you use it to *think*. That's not meant to be insulting; it's an absolutely critical truth for those who can accept and embrace it. Our society has become so compartmentalized, specialized, industrialized, and socialized that people are used to outsourcing virtually every decision in every area of their lives.

Sink stopped up? Call the plumber. Car running rough? Ring the mechanic. Not feeling well? Go to the doctor.

At times, that's fine – necessary, even. But those who rely entirely on others get taken advantage of, and typically obtain a much lower level of service. To get the most from others, you need to know what you're doing.

And there's one more point, as well. If you pay close attention as you try new therapies, you'll be able to detect increasingly minute reactions in your body. Your ability to perceive very small reactions – good and bad – will steadily and greatly increase. And when you try a new exercise and it causes pain, you'll know to avoid that exercise, procedure, technique, or treatment.

It's almost impossible to overemphasize the importance of this perceptivity. When we're healthy and strong, we can be incredibly insensitive to our body's response to stimuli. We can sustain damage for a long time before the pain becomes enough to get our attention. But if you bring this attitude to a healing situation, you'll miss a great deal of absolutely crucial information your body is imparting. Worse, you could exacerbate the injury.

I provide this warning especially for those who were taught to ignore pain in order to accomplish their goals. Such training is often good for life, but it's bad for healing. Having played college football and gone through airborne and ranger training in the Army, I know all about such a mindset. Had I given way to every ache and pain, I would never have completed my first day of training. But when my back eventually gave way to years of abuse and I had to stop relentlessly hard-charging, I found that ignoring pain didn't give me the information I needed to deal with my recuperation.

My back problem is a severe one, and it has taken years to treat. Health professionals have given me scores of exercises to help it heal properly. I've learned that, generally speaking, the ones that make me feel better are good, and the ones that make me feel worse are bad. Sounds like a no-brainer, right? It's not. Some of the differences in feeling are so minute that in my earlier days, when most of my training hurt *a lot*, I wouldn't have given it a second thought. If the "expert" told me to do it, it must be good for me. Never mind the pain, just do it.

Now I know that even small benefits I get from an exercise can be built on to increase strength and flexibility. Conversely, if the impact is small but adverse, I know not to do the exercise anymore. Over time, the impact will become serious. That, I don't need. (This applies to habits, too, not just exercises – habits such as sitting and standing properly, eating well, and not allowing stress to build up.)

So learn to pay attention to the small things, and to direct your own recovery. No one can discern the impact of treatment on your body as well as you can, so don't cede authority for your treatment to anyone else. They're only advisors. You must be in charge of your healing, and the more you know about the human body, your particular injury or illness, various treatment options, and the reaction of your body to various stimuli, the better you will do.

The Individuality of Wellness ... and Pain ... and Treatment

One of the nice things about natural (or alternative) medicine is that it typically has a very limited downside. Most natural treatments have very little potential for harm. Because of this fact, for over two decades of researching and writing in the medical field, I have made myself a continual guinea pig. You name it – vitamins, minerals, diets, detox protocols, acupuncture, prolotherapy, ultraviolet blood irradiation, oxygen therapies, and much more – I've tried it. I needed to know the therapies I was writing about or recommending were safe.

But I couldn't always use my experiences as a good assessment of efficacy. Why not? Because few therapies, natural or otherwise, affect all people the same way. Even the best therapies often cure significantly less than 100 percent of those who try them. Medical studies invariably assess efficacy in terms of percentages of participants who respond favorably. And success is often measured in surprisingly low percentages, depending on the intractability of the condition being treated.

All of which is to say that, when it comes to medicine, there are – and *must* be – different strokes for different folks. People vary to an amazing degree in their physiological and psychological makeup. What works for one *often* doesn't work for another. So if something I recommend in this report doesn't work for you, don't get angry. Try another therapy. If that doesn't work, try again.

That can be frustrating, I know. I've done it – many times. The time, the expense, the disappointment – they can wear you down. But don't despair, and don't give up. This is a necessary part of developing your most important tool for dealing with pain – your mind. Even failures will help you toward your goal if you learn from them. They will tell you things that, taken together, will *often* help you succeed in the end. Don't stop trying, and above all don't stop *thinking*.

Most people will have bought this report hoping for a magic bullet to cure their pain. I don't say that condescendingly; I know because I buy reports for that purpose, too. But it seldom happens. Things that work usually *take* work. So the temptation is to set the report aside and look for the next big promise.

But this report summarizes the results of hundreds of thousands of hours of work, study, research, and treatment. The potential is here for you to learn much not only about curing pain, but about how your body works, how your mind works, and even how human nature works. Those things are worth learning, and they greatly contribute to success. I've been told that Thomas Edison once said, "I didn't fail, I just found 10,000 things that didn't work." Yet today we know him for his successes – *hundreds* of them. Really important successes. Because he kept trying, learned from his mistakes and failures, and used his head. The same process will work for all of us.

Chapter 2

How to Get the Right Help
When Going It Alone Isn't Enough

This is a bit of a counterintuitive section. Most people who order reports like this one are both highly capable and very independent. Many find that "professionals" are seldom as good as they ought to be. Other readers are constrained by cost. Still others put more store in their own counsel than anyone else's. I get all that. This report will give you a great deal to work with if that's your bent (which I assume it is; it's certainly mine).

But the point still needs to be made that two heads are often better than one. America has always produced more than its share of innovative, conscientious, competent professionals – in just about every field. That's certainly been true in medicine. And it's an important fact you'll need to take advantage of as you deal with your pain and any future health issues that may arise.

America's healthcare system is an industrialized one – a system that turns the giving of the most basic of healthcare into a complex protocol involving multiple people with high-level degrees, untold regulations, third-party payers (insurers and government benefit programs), reams of paperwork, scores of medical studies, and further complications beyond belief. It is badly broken. But a couple of folksy aphorisms apply: Even a blind hog finds an occasional acorn. And help is where you find it. Within this massive, bureaucratic, industrial machine we call American healthcare, there are a few exceptional people who regularly transcend their professions. If you turn your back on them because they are part of a broken, exploitative system, you will miss out on help that might make the difference for you.

This underscores the need to find good people ahead of time. One of the biggest reasons alternative health care lovers (and others, too, for that matter) get hurt by the conventional medical system is because they sustain a major injury or have a serious health incident and have to go see a doctor. They don't like the medical system, so they don't have a doctor they trust in such a crucial time. They're at the mercy of whomever they can find. Perhaps they have to go to the emergency room because they don't have anyone else who deals with urgent health issues. "The system" takes over, they become pawns in the game, and many of the things they've learned to avoid over the years are foisted on them because the perceived (and perhaps real) alternative is death or serious disability.

If you've taken the time to find good medical professionals ahead of time, you can call on them in times of emergency. They can help you with critical decisions and offer you alternatives that can even help in the hospital. You'll have options and allies, and those are very good things to have.

When looking for such allies, look for someone who regularly transcends their training. Whether they've been trained traditionally or alternatively, anyone who does only what they've been taught is a disaster waiting to happen. Medicine is far too complex to practice by rote or by recipe. It's a thinking person's profession. Make sure you look for people who can and will think, and who can and will act independently of the *immense* peer pressure so prevalent in the health field. Look also for people who have a "gift" for healing (people who have both intuition and skill for finding and effectively treating the problem), and who have personal concern for the people they treat.

If you find such a person – or a number of them – make good use of them and *hold on to them*. They are the true healers. There are not many of them, and they are in great demand.

The best way to find such professionals is by personal recommendations from people you trust who have personal experience with the professionals being recommended. Start a bulletin board or booklet featuring recommended professionals at your place of work or among friends or within a group you're a member of. Actively solicit people's recommendations, with supporting comments. Such items are extremely helpful. If you're not a good networker, befriend someone who is. You can also get some information online, but that's a tougher area. You don't know the reliability of the person making the recommendation, so you'll have to be very discerning. That source can still be helpful, however.

Kinds of Pain, and What Each One Needs to Make It Go Away

In this section, we'll conduct a brief analysis of the types of problems that cause some of the more common, widespread kinds of pain. Major treatments will be described in later chapters, while some of the minor, more specific therapies will be included here. If your source of pain is not mentioned here by name, you may still find help within these descriptions. If the source of your pain (nerves, muscles, inflammation, etc.) is similar to conditions described here, you can often benefit from treatments shown to be beneficial for similar conditions.

Chapter 3

Arthritis and Other
Inflammation-related Pain

Arthritis is caused by inflammation. You might not be familiar with inflammation as a cause of disease, but you're almost certainly aware of inflammation as a bodily response to injury. If you've ever had a twisted knee, a jammed finger, or a sprained ankle, you know that the tissues surrounding the injury swell, heat up, turn red, and produce pain. Your ability to use the injured body part is often greatly reduced, as well. These reactions typically speed healing, even as they inhibit you from using the problem area and further injuring it.

Like pain itself, as long as inflammation does its job and goes away, it's a good thing. But if inflammation becomes chronic – it just won't leave – the situation is much different. Arthritis is a problem precisely because of this long-term aspect of its nature. It is one of the most familiar forms of chronic inflammation (cardiovascular disease, asthma, and chronic obstructive pulmonary disease [COPD] are others, but though extremely serious they are not necessarily painful). Other painful inflammatory diseases include lupus and eczema. Though the body is trying to deal with what it perceives as a threat, its response soon becomes as bad as or worse than the threat.

In treating arthritis pain, modern medicine has done us a huge disservice. Many of the drugs most commonly used to treat it actually increase the degeneration of cartilage in the joints. This further increases the pain, and significantly worsens the joint injury. Clinical trials have demonstrated that the class of pain-relieving drugs known as nonsteroidal anti-inflammatory drugs (NSAIDs) inhibits the body's repair processes, which in turn leads to breakdown in the articular (joint) cartilage. NSAIDS can especially affect hip and knee joints. Aspirin, ibuprofen, celecoxib, and naproxen are among the many drugs that can cause this serious problem.[1]

Arthritis is fairly easy to self-diagnose, but particularly if you're female and elderly, and your pain is in the small joints of your hands and feet, you might want to get a professional diagnosis. These conditions are more likely to indicate rheumatoid arthritis, and time is of the essence in treating this condition. It is a fast-developing disease, and typically deforms the joints permanently. It's nothing to ignore or treat casually, and rheumatoid arthritis differs in its cause

1   *Newman NM, et al. Acetabular bone destruction related to non-steroidal anti-inflammatory drugs. Lancet. July 6,1985:11-13.*

Huskisson HC, et al. Effects of anti-inflammatory drugs on the progression of osteoarthritis of the knee. Journal of Rheumatology. 1995;(22):1941-1946.

Reijman M, et al. Is there an association between the use of different types of nonsteroidal anti-inflammatory drugs and radiologic progression of osteoarthritis? The Rotterdam Study. Arthritis & Rheumatism. 2005;(52):3137-3142.

and treatment from osteoarthritis (though, as you'll see, a number of treatments are effective for both).

Osteoarthritis

Osteoarthritis is the most common form of arthritis. Many people refer to it as "wear and tear" arthritis because it comes from physical activity that literally wears down or tears apart the cartilage that protects bones from bearing on one another. As this buffering, lubricating layer of cartilage disintegrates, the friction and impact of the bones on each other and nearby soft tissues causes tissue damage and resultant inflammation. When you have osteoarthritis, this is what you're feeling. This form of arthritis is more common in major joints such as knee, hip, and back, though it certainly affects smaller joints, such as those in the hands, as well.

By far the most important and efficacious means of dealing with osteoarthritis is via proper nutrition. It's also the hardest thing for many people to do. I wish I could change that because better nutrition would not only relieve the arthritis suffering of tens of millions of people, it would improve the health of hundreds of millions. Nutrition is fully that powerful. But Americans love their junk food, comfort food, stress-relief food, desserts, and traditional food. It's an emotional thing, not a contemplative one. And emotions are powerful things.

In addition to (or even in lieu of) good nutrition, several of the therapies I'll mention in a moment are extremely helpful for osteoarthritis. Some of them result in complete cures for many people, and frequently offer major relief to those they do not cure. But the fact remains that the most potent means of dealing with osteoarthritis is through nutrition. You'll read about nutrition's benefits in Chapter 7. Even if eating right is very difficult for you, I encourage you to read the chapter and think about it. Then keep reading about nutrition. Over time, you'll begin to effect a change in your thinking that will help you implement the necessary changes in your diet. Most healthy eaters didn't develop their mindsets on nutrition overnight.

Because osteoarthritis is due to damage in the joints, therapies that are able to target the joints can be very helpful. Prolotherapy can be very helpful here, as can prolozone®. These therapies use substances that are injected near the site of the damage, and help the body repair injured tissue. Both can be highly efficacious, though prolozone is typically faster-acting than prolotherapy. They are explained at length in Chapter 13.

Topical therapies such as essential oils and DMSO can afford some rapid, temporary relief. These are typically substances that you either rub or massage into the skin surrounding the affected area. Chapter 9 details which oils to use and how to use them.

Oxygen therapies can be very helpful for osteoarthritis, and include hydrogen peroxide therapy, exercise with oxygen therapy, and hyperbaric oxygen therapy. By providing oxygen to oxygen-poor joints, each of these therapies can provide not only relief, but often repair of injured tissues. You'll read about them in Chapter 12, along with how critical oxygen is to the repair and even rebuilding of injured tissues.

In the chapter on light therapy (Chapter 10), you'll read how John Ott cured his arthritis with sunlight. Simply taking ambient (not direct) sunlight in through his eyes made such a difference that he was able to stop using his cane to walk. If that sounds incredible to you, you'll definitely want to read the whole chapter on light therapy. It's not as far-fetched as it might seem at first. Mr. Ott does not specify the type of arthritis he had, but I suspect it was osteoarthritis (it was in his hip). Sunlight is the ultimate in simple, inexpensive (free), pleasant, efficacious medicine.

Several other forms of light therapy have also had positive effects on osteoarthritis. These include color therapy, polarized light therapy, and laser therapy, all detailed in Chapter 10.

Magnetic therapies have been demonstrated to have positive effects on osteoarthritis. Both permanent magnets and pulsed electromagnetic field (PEMF) therapy can be effective. PEMF tends to deal more effectively with chronic pain, which is what osteoarthritis typically is, but permanent magnets can offer significant relief as well. These therapies are described in Chapter 11.

Rheumatoid Arthritis

Rheumatoid arthritis (RA) is referred to as an "autoimmune disease." What this means in the mainstream view is that the body's immune system attacks the lining in the joints, causing painful swelling. Some doctors disagree with this characterization, saying RA is instead caused by an infection.[2] This is why, they posit, the antibiotic minocycline is often highly effective in treating RA. As an alternative to antibiotics, you can often get similar effects with prolozone. Because of the antimicrobial nature of ozone, this therapy kills many infections even as it stimulates healing and regrowth of bodily tissues. You can read more about prolozone in Chapter 13.

Vitamin D is also extremely helpful in dealing with rheumatoid arthritis – as it is with several autoimmune diseases, including multiple sclerosis and insulin dependent diabetes.[3] You can up your vitamin D levels by spending more time in the sun (indirect sun is sufficient if you are light skinned), by eating more oily fish or cod liver oil, or by direct supplementation. If you take supplemental vitamin D, therapeutic levels for those who are deficient in D are 4,000-6,000 IU per day.[4]

Be careful if you choose to use fish products to up your vitamin D levels. Many fish and fish-oil products contain high levels of mercury, which worsens RA. Use only products or fish

2   Rowen R. Antibiotic prevents Parkinson's. *Second Opinion.* 2002;12(9).
3   Rowen R. This free nutrient works wonders. *Second Opinion.* 2002;12(10).
4   Ibid.

that are known to be mercury free or have very low levels.

Because mercury and other heavy metals greatly exacerbate the onset and symptoms of RA, chelation therapy can be helpful. This therapy will be discussed in greater detail later in this chapter, but its essence is this: Heavy metals tend to accumulate in the organs rather than being excreted from the body. This includes the brain. Hat makers of old, who used mercuric nitrate in the making of felt hats, tended to show eccentric behavior after a while because of this tendency. They had high brain mercury levels, and were prone to becoming "mad hatters." In order to remove the metals from the body, a substance must be used that binds to the metals and causes the body to excrete them. This is what chelation agents do. Using them can significantly reduce levels of heavy metals in the body, which in turn can greatly aid in the treatment of RA.

A form of light therapy that has been effective for RA is ultraviolet blood irradiation (UBI), described in Chapter 10. This therapy greatly strengthens the immune system, giving credence to the infection theory of RA (if it were truly an autoimmune disease, strengthening the immune system would worsen the problem, not improve it).

Color therapy has also been effective in the treatment of RA. Other light therapy options include polarized light therapy and laser therapy. These therapies are all also described in Chapter 10.

Topically, essential oils and DMSO have proved useful for RA pain. They are described in Chapter 9. Both light therapy and topical therapy should be used as supplemental therapies to faster-acting therapies such as prolozone, UBI, pulsed electromagnetic field therapy, or even antibiotics if you're so inclined. Light and topical therapies are useful (and light therapy *can* be [and often is] quick and curative for major health problems), but this disease must be authoritatively dealt with before it can deform the joints permanently.

Pulsed electromagnetic field, or PEMF, therapy has also proved effective in the treatment of RA. As the name implies, this is an electromagnetic field therapy that operates on a pulsed electrical current. You can read about this powerful treatment in Chapter 11.

The oxygenation therapies have proved effective for RA, including hydrogen peroxide therapy, exercise with oxygen therapy, and hyperbaric oxygen therapy. These therapies are described at greater length in Chapter 12. They, too, should probably be used supplementally with some of the faster-acting therapies mentioned above.

Other Inflammation-Related Conditions

Inflammation-related pain in general is so widespread that it cannot be responsibly covered in a report this size. However, most forms of such pain fall into three categories: injury, infection, and autoimmune disease, the first two of which have been or will be covered here and the third of which we will discuss in a few instances. Obviously, there is some overlap between these categories: RA may be an autoimmune disease or an infection, infection can cause injury to tissues, etc. But we'll use these categories as broadly useful designations nonetheless. If the doctor who diagnoses your inflammation-related source of pain can describe its nature for you, you can then apply some of the therapies appropriate to that kind of pain.

With injuries, the cause is often easy to identify. And with common, non-catastrophic injuries, the healing process is usually pretty straightforward and unproblematic. It's when you're dealing with a catastrophic injury or a chronic irritant that the issue gets a bit more difficult.

Inflammation will continue to occur in injured tissues, so severe injuries pose particular problems. Because the physiology of the body has been altered, either the alteration itself or the resultant altered function of the body cause continued inflammation, and often continued pain. Manipulative therapies such as massage or chiropractic can often restore sufficient physiological normalcy to reduce or eliminate the pain, but in severe cases something more is required. Reconstructive surgery is often the only course of action that can restore a sufficient level of physiological normalcy (though that is often very difficult, given the complexity of the body), and thus provide some relief from the body's overambitious inflammatory attempts to heal itself.

Lifestyle modification may also be called for – and is one of the most difficult things for many people to do. People typically want their former lives back, and some injuries make that impossible. Making the transition to new habits and new interests can be one of the hardest – and most rewarding – things you'll ever do. No longer doing activities that exacerbate the injury, finding things that help it heal (such as a better mattress, chair, or workstation), pursuing new interests that don't aggravate the injury (but may help you develop new abilities), and learning to focus on more important things than the pain can all make a world of difference when you're faced with an intractable source of pain.

Another cause of injury-related chronic inflammation is the presence of some irritant within the body. The irritant can be a toxic substance, such as a chemical or a heavy metal; it can be a problem food (usually one of your habitual favorites); it can be an allergen; or it can even (apparently) be some element of the body itself – resulting in an autoimmune response. Because the irritant persists within the body, the body continues to respond to the irritant with inflammation. Thus, in the case of non-autoimmune irritants, the key to success is to identify and remove the source of the irritation. And in the case of autoimmune irritants, the key is to pacify as much as possible the body's immune response. (As mentioned earlier, autoimmune diseases are greatly exacerbated by the presence of heavy metals, so the question is open as to whether the body is actually acting against itself or is acting against toxic elements absorbed in bodily tissues – or perhaps against tissues damaged or altered by such elements.)

For most irritants, diagnosis is the key – and the hardest thing to do. That might sound like a truism because diagnosis is often both key and difficult for many health problems. But in this case it's particularly problematic – for the simple reason that modern society and modern medicine have defined as harmless many things we take into our bodies that are potentially harmful: mercury from dental fillings, chlorine and fluoride from municipal water supplies, artificial sweeteners in our food, as well as simple carbohydrates (especially sugar), food preservatives, a host of unpronounceable food additives, genetically modified organisms (GMOs), and scores of chemicals we absorb through our skin from soaps and shampoos, beauty products, insecticides and herbicides, household cleaning products, clothing and linen, and mattresses (which, by law – at the instigation of chemical manufacturers – must now be treated with toxic chemical flame retardants that absorb into the skin).

Some of these substances may be benign or nearly so. Many are far from it. The problem is that efforts to determine the exact level of hazard they pose are routinely thwarted by parties that have a financial stake in their sale. The products that contain these substances represent many billions of dollars in sales every year. And many businesspeople seem to care more about customers' money than their health.

The point here is not to be negative. It is simply to point out that these substances commonly regarded as benign, or at least minimally toxic, can be sources of injury to your bodily tissues, and thereby trigger an inflammation response in your body. If you want to be free of your inflammation and its consequent pain, you must be free of the substance or substances that are causing it. Find out what it is (or they are) and you're more than half way there.

Most doctors are minimally helpful in this regard. Many do not regard the toxins we face as problems. Some regard every toxin you've ever encountered as a poison that's about to kill you. Finding someone with the understanding both that toxins are dangerous and that some are worse than others is difficult.[5] But there are doctors who specialize in this kind of thing (see the Resource section for doctors who specialize in environmental medicine).

Once known, the sources of your inflammation can often be removed. By far the most common problem is substances that come from your diet. Foods have an amazing ability to cause the body harm, even as they are essential for life. In short, nutrition is exceptionally powerful – for good or for ill. And the likelihood that nutrition can address your inflammation-related problem is very high. Chapter 7 will detail many of the nutritional steps you can take to reduce or eliminate your inflammation-related pain.

If the source of your inflammation is more toxic, in the form of chemical or heavy metal exposure and absorption, you'll need to detoxify your body. This can be done in a few different ways. Start with a high-fiber, low-simple carb, diet. This should increase your eliminations to one

---

5   One example, though not technically a toxin, is radon. Many people think that radon exposure will destroy their health and kill them. That's like saying water will kill you. The statement contains an element of truth, but the devil's in the details. Many places that humans inhabit have ambient levels of radiation that come from the earth. We thrive on them because the body has defenses against low-level radiation that are kept in shape by exposure (a concept called "hormesis" – small amounts of harmful substances are good for us because they enhance our resistance to them). Problems arise only when levels get too high. Many homebuilding regulations recognize this reality, but many people who write or advise on the subject medically or environmentally do not.

to three times a day, which is a natural and effective way to detox. If that doesn't do the trick, you might be dealing with heavy metal poisoning. A hair tissue mineral analysis can tell you if this is the case (doctors can order this for you, or you can order one directly online). If it is, you're probably a candidate for chelation therapy. This involves infusing a chelation agent intravenously. The agent binds to heavy metals and allows your body to excrete them. You can find a chelation practitioner near you by going to the American College for Advancement in Medicine Web site at acamnet.org and clicking on "Find a Physician in Your Area" at the bottom of the page under "Public Information."

You might also need to have amalgam fillings removed from your teeth, as these fillings contain high levels of mercury (they are approximately 50 percent mercury). This cannot be done casually, as drilling out the amalgam fillings without protecting the patient can greatly increase mercury exposure rather than decrease it. If your dentist is not well versed in this sensitive procedure, you can find one who is by looking on the Web site of the International Academy of Biological Dentistry & Medicine at http://biologicaldentistrydirectory.com; the Holistic Dental Association, holisticdental.org/find_holistic_dentist; or the International Association of Mercury Free Dentists, https://dentalwellness4u.hostasaurus.com/freeservices/find_dentists.html.

If your mercury levels are already high and you don't have ready access to intravenous chelation therapy, you might want to consider an oral chelation agent (a chelation agent taken by mouth, as a pill). Oral chelators have always been regarded as far less effective than IV chelators, but that might be changing. Hungarian researchers have found that a product made from peat chelates mercury even better than intravenous chelation.[6,7] Over the course of their 11-day study, the peat complex increased mercury elimination by 21 percent. Further, and even more importantly, mercury in the brain was reduced by 87 percent over that seen in the study controls. This is very high-level effectiveness. Metal Magnet from Enzymatic Therapies, enzy.com, is one product that makes use of this discovery.

Another crucial advance in battling inflammation was made by researchers working jointly from Mount Sinai University and China. They used a mix of Chinese herbs they called antiasthma herbal medicine intervention, or ASHMI. In the study they conducted on 91 asthma patients, they tested this herbal combination against 20 mg prednisone tablets and a placebo designed to look like the prednisone tablets.[8] Prednisone is a steroid, and is the treatment of choice for the kind of inflammation presented by asthma. However, it tends to reduce the adrenal gland's ability to make hormones so badly that the effects can last for years.

Asthma patients tend to be very low in cortisol, a natural steroid produced within the body that helps control inflammation. The study participants were found to exhibit this condition.

6   Rashad S, Revell P, Hemingway A, et al. *Effect of non-steroidal anti-inflammatory drugs on the course of osteo-arthritis. Lancet. 1989;(2):519-522.*

7   Department of Biochemistry, University of Kapsovar, Kapsovar, Hungary.

8   Wen MC, Wei CH, Hu ZQ, et al. Efficacy and tolerability of antiasthma herbal medicine intervention in adult patients with moderate-severe allergic asthma. *J Allergy Clin Immunol* 2005;116(3):517-524.

The prednisone and ASHMI groups exhibited a significant improvement in lung function over the course of the study. Though the prednisone group had slightly better results in that regard, the group members experienced a decrease in cortisol from their already depressed levels. However, the ASHMI group members experienced a significant increase in cortisol levels.

The importance of this finding, and the reason it is included here, though asthma is not generally characterized by excessive pain, is that a dietary supplement that can increase the body's cortisol levels safely and naturally holds great promise for treating other inflammatory conditions. If you suffer from a painful inflammatory disease, it is definitely an option you should consider. The herbal combination contains reishi (*Ganoderma lucidum*), shrubby sophora (*Sophora flavescens*), Chinese licorice (*Glycyrrhiza uralensis*), and noni (*Morinda citrifolia*). You can get it in a product called PhytoCort® at allergyresearchgroup.com.

To further deal with the pain associated with inflammation-related problems, some of the therapies mentioned in the next section (Injury-related Pain) can be helpful. Particularly, topical treatments such as DMSO or essential oils can be helpful. Light therapy can also be quite helpful. These therapies can be studied at greater length in Chapters 9 and 10, respectively. With inflammation-related pain, however, the only lasting relief you'll find will be in removing or correcting the source of injury to your body's susceptible tissues.

Chapter 4

Injury-related Pain

Your nerve cells are made so they are nonresponsive (not transmitting pain – or pleasure, for that matter) only when they're undisturbed. When a detrimental change in your body's physiology occurs, they begin transmitting pain signals to your cortex. That change can be a cut, an impact, a shift in your physiology caused by strong forces (whiplash from a car accident, for example), excessive heat or cold, an adverse chemical reaction, inflammation, and so forth. All of these changes threaten the integrity of your bodily structures, so your nerve cells tell you about that. And when bad things happen, the language they speak is pain.

Unfortunately, nerves don't accommodate themselves to permanent changes in your body from injury. They don't get used to the "new normal" and stop telling you about it. To the degree that your body heals and reestablishes the old normal, the nerves will quiet down. But if there are vestiges of the injury that remain, your nerves will tell you all about it, repeatedly, insistently, continuously. This is a major reason Bayer has been a very lucrative company for well over a hundred years.

So with an injury, the best thing you can do is to reestablish the old normal as soon and as completely as you can. If you have a catastrophic injury, where parts of your body have been broken or shattered, it's time to call on your network of hyper-competent healers. Those are certainly cases where experts are required.

Most injuries are not so catastrophic, however, and there's a great deal you can do on your own to reestablish normal physiology. We'll spend most of the rest of this report in this area, since this is where most readers will likely want the most information.

For most such injuries to peripheral areas (arms and legs, including shoulders and hips), you'll want to greatly reduce the use of the affected body part (if it hurts, "don't do that"). This means taking all strain and most weight-bearing off of it. The use of splints and slings can be useful, but total immobilization is not advised unless the injury is severe (in which case you should be taking your hyper-competent doctor's advice, not mine). The injury will heal faster and better if some use is maintained, along with using the limb throughout whatever range of motion does not produce pain (increase the range of motion as healing allows).

To reduce the pain as healing occurs, consider several options:

Topical treatments are a good place to start if the injury is not severe. These treatments are described in greater depth in Chapter 9, but here are some products you should consider. DMSO is a great place to start. It's inexpensive, readily available, deep penetrating, and highly effective at relieving many kinds of pain. Just be sure to observe the cautions listed in the longer write-up on topical treatments.

Many essential oils have pain-relieving properties, as well. They can be a bit on the expensive side, but a little goes a long way – and they're much cheaper than a trip to the doctor's office. With essential oils, you can effectively create your own pharmacy, with which you can efficaciously treat a large array of health challenges – far beyond pain relief.

Treatments that use some form of electromagnetic radiation can be very helpful in relieving pain. These include various forms of light therapy, such as colored light therapy, polarized light therapy, and laser therapy. Other forms of electromagnetic therapy include the use of therapeutic magnets and PEMF therapy. Some of these therapies are among the least expensive you'll ever find. Others entail an initial outlay for a device, and are thereafter virtually free. These treatments, and the devices they require, are described in Chapter 10.

Oxygen therapies can also be extremely helpful for healing injuries – especially joint injuries. Joints are not well served by arterial blood supply, as the cartilage, tendons, and ligaments that comprise them do not require as much oxygen in normal operation as blood and bone do. When injured, though, these tissues require significant increases in oxygen to heal. The inflammation that accompanies an injury accomplishes some of this increase in oxygenation, but anything you can do to further saturate the injured tissues with oxygen will speed the process of healing. Oxygen therapies do precisely this, so they can at times produce significant increases in the rate of healing. Some of the most useful oxygen therapies include the use of a hyperbaric oxygen chamber, exercise with oxygen therapy, and intravenous hydrogen peroxide therapy. See Chapter 12 for more details.

Another particularly helpful family of therapies for joint injuries is that of the prolotherapies. These include prolotherapy and prolozone (prolozone is also something of an oxygen therapy, since the ozone injected into the body breaks down into oxygen). The theory behind these therapies is fascinating, as is their ability to hasten the healing of several types of injuries. All this is detailed in Chapter 13.

Other helpful therapies also require experts to administer them, but ought not to be written off if you have the means to avail yourself of them. Two areas that have seen great advances in innovation and efficacy are massage therapy and physical therapy. Both are characterized by high numbers of extremely competent practitioners. I have been amazed by the number of good ones I have either gone to or heard or read about over the past decade or two. Both of these therapies can reduce pain and convalescence times significantly.

Which brings us to the other professions that employ manipulation of the body to restore normal alignment and function: osteopathy and chiropractic. These professions, too, have seen radical improvements in knowledge and skill related to their field of expertise. Anyone who saw a chiropractor in the 1960s or '70s would be simply amazed at the increased sophistication and efficacy of treatment today. I say this from personal experience. The difference is truly astounding.

The field of chiropractic has exploded both in breadth and depth. Whole new fields have opened up (there are at least 20 available now), incorporating vast new knowledge of human physiology and interrelationships within the body. Connections that were not even suspected before are now common knowledge. For instance, during a recent bout of back trouble, I experienced severe pain in my left thigh and on the outside of my left upper leg and knee. This pain was actually being caused by compression of a nerve in the lumbar region of my back. To relieve my leg pain, the chiropractor adjusted the L3/L4 region of my back (the third and fourth lumbar vertebrae), which worked every time.

This can be a bit strange. I would go into the chiropractor with intolerable pain in my leg, and he would start to work on my back. He hardly touched my leg. I wondered if he knew what he was doing until the pain in my leg went away (temporarily, it turned out, but unmistakably and therapeutically – it got better after doing this over time). This is high-level understanding of physiology and the interrelationships (of which there are many) between seemingly unrelated parts of the body.

Osteopaths have made similar advances in understanding the body's physiology, and have the benefit of access to all aspects of conventional medicine, when that's appropriate or necessary. Osteopaths are essentially medical doctors – plus. They are trained in the same disciplines as M.D.s, but are also trained in manipulation of the musculoskeletal system. Thus, they can make better use of the most direct application of hand-eye-brain coordination.

Therapeutically, hands are astonishingly capable tools. They can find and treat a multitude of problems. A person who knows what a joint should feel and act like can quickly see what the problem is when it goes off the rails. And he or she can often put it back into correct alignment so it can function correctly either immediately or with several treatments that keep things lined up while healing occurs. They can also cause over-tight muscles to relax, thus relieving pressure on joints. Moreover, if you pay attention to what they're doing, you can often do a lesser and more gentle version of their manipulations on yourself or your family at home.

During a recent spate of back problems, I paid close attention to how my back was adjusted at the doctor's office. When I got home, my wife offered to help and I told her how and where to massage (not adjust) or put pressure on my back in key places I had learned from the doctor. By having her do that every day, sometimes multiple times a day, I was able to extend the time between doctor visits by as much as several weeks.

Zero balancing and craniosacral therapy are extremely therapeutic manipulation techniques. They, along with Bowen therapy and pain neutralization technique are explained in Chapter 14.

At this point in this chapter, I'd like to challenge your thinking with something of a counterintuitive concept. We're used to thinking of injury as I have described it thus far, but there is another condition we don't think of as an injury that nonetheless acts on the body in an injurious fashion. I'm talking about obesity – excess weight. An injury alters the function of the body, sometimes a little, sometimes a lot. So does obesity.

You may have observed the difference in a person's gait and movements that occurs as they gain weight. They tend to hold back their upper torso to counterbalance their abdominal weight, thus overarching and stressing the lower back, and they walk with more of a diagonal gait (legs moving forward and out with each step) than one that moves straight forward and back in the line of travel. This stresses all of the leg joints from the hip to the ankle. The axis along which a joint moves can be altered by weight, and the load the joint is carrying can also be increased. Precisely as happens with an injury, the normal operation of the body has been altered.

The combination of altered range of movement and increased load can be quite injurious to a joint. If you like dark meat in a chicken, consider how you separate the leg from the thigh when you want to eat them separately. You might twist the joint and apply force (pull). This combination usually does the trick, separating the two pieces at the joint. This is an exaggeration of what happens in the obese body, but it is accurate in concept (pushing on the joint is less damaging than pulling on it, but is still quite injurious when it involves excess forces).

In the case of obesity, the cure is simpler – which is not to say easier – than with most injuries. Just lose the weight. This can be very hard for some people, but the stakes are high – this could be the difference between a life of pain and a pain-free life. See Chapter 7 on nutrition and Chapter 8 on exercise for some crucial information on how to accomplish this important goal.

Chapter 5

Nerve-related Pain

A significant source of sometimes excruciating pain can be nerve-related pain. That figures, of course. Nerves relay pain, so anything that targets or affects them directly is bound to be instantly felt and high on the pain scale. Such maladies can include peripheral neuropathy, shingles, and fibromyalgia (possibly – fibromyalgia's exact cause and nature is a matter of some uncertainty and speculation; it is typically, however, characterized as a neurosensory disorder).

Peripheral Neuropathy

Peripheral neuropathy is caused by damage to the nerves, and results in numbness or pain in the hands or feet. Its causes are many, so treatment is often quite varied, as well. But some of the more common causes are diabetes, age, genetic predisposition, toxins, excessive alcohol intake, nutritional deficiencies – particularly of B vitamins, or as a drug side effect (including statins).

The place to start with this problem is with the dietary supplement alpha lipoic acid (ALA), particularly if the problem is due to diabetes. A study published in a Chinese journal followed 95 type-2 diabetic patients, divided into two groups.[9] One group received 600 mg of ALA intravenously once a day for 14 days. The other group received a placebo. The results were significant and were seen after only one week. Over 90 percent of the ALA group improved vs. only 14 percent in the placebo group.

Another study showed an even more stark contrast.[10] It involved oral ingestion of 600 mg of ALA daily for six months. Nearly 77 percent of the recipients experienced a complete clearing of all their symptoms. Not one person in either group had any side effects.

Dr. Frank Shallenberger has had at least one non-diabetic, elderly patient respond to ALA, so this supplement is not limited to treating neuropathy caused by diabetes. Age-related neuropathy also responds to this treatment. ALA may work because it stimulates the production of nitric oxide in the body, which is in short supply in both diabetics and the elderly. But if ALA doesn't work, other options that have proved to help peripheral neuropathy include: topical capsaicin (cayenne pepper), vitamin E, glutathione, folic acid, vitamin B6, biotin, myo-inositol,

9   Liu F, Zhang M, Yang B, et al. Curative effect of alpha-lipoic acid on peripheral neuropathy in type-2 diabetes: a clinical study. *Zhonghua Yi Xue Za Zhi.* 2007;87(38);2706-2709. Cited by Shallenberger F. Peripheral neuropathy cured in seven days. *Real Cures.* 2007;10(2):1-5.

10   Negrianu G, Ro M, Bolte UB, Lefter D, Dabelea D. Effects of three-month treatment with the antioxidant alpha-lipoic acid in diabetic peripheral neuropathy. *Rom J Intern Med.* 1999;37(3):297-306. Cited by Shallenberger. Peripheral neuropathy cured in seven days: 3.

fish oil, L-arginine, L-glutamine, taurine, N-acetylcysteine, zinc, magnesium, chromium, St. John's wort, acupuncture, magnetic therapy, and infrared laser therapy.[11]

Another study on diabetic neuropathy gave one of three groups in the 75-person study zinc (20 mg), magnesium (250 mg), vitamin C (200 mg), and vitamin E (100 mg) each day for four months. The participants experienced a 75 percent decrease in their neuropathic symptoms. A second group that was given this same regimen along with the B vitamins B1 (10 mg), B2 (10 mg), B6 (200 µg), B12 (10 µg), and folic acid (1 mg) saw their symptom scores fall from 3.45 to 0.64. These are clearly some micronutrients that you should try if you are suffering from diabetic neuropathy.

Shingles

Shingles is a form of herpes, like cold sores. It's caused by the outbreak of a variant form of the chickenpox virus, Herpes varicella zoster. Those who have had chickenpox in the past might have the herpes zoster virus lying dormant within their bodies. High levels of physical or emotional stress can be the necessary trigger to cause an outbreak, especially if the immune system is compromised. Many people describe it as the worst pain they've ever experienced, so you need a better plan than to "grit your teeth and bear it."

If you start to come down with shingles, try intravenous vitamin C, ultraviolet radiation therapy (Chapter 10), intravenous hydrogen peroxide (Chapter 12), or ozone. Up to 5,000 IU of vitamin D daily should also be of help.[12]

You might also try some essential oils, including lemon balm. Mix a few drops with a little bit of olive oil and use it topically on the affected areas. You could also try a few drops in an ointment. Other essential oils that have antiviral properties include lavender, eucalyptus, oregano, chamomile, tea tree, and sage. Each should be mixed with a carrier oil such as olive oil (typically one to five drops of essential oil to one teaspoon of carrier oil) to keep the essential oil from burning the skin. Ravenserra has been found to be effective in treating shingles, as well.[13]

Fibromyalgia

Fibromyalgia has been hard to define in the past, but is now defined by the Mayo Clinic as "a disorder characterized by widespread musculoskeletal pain accompanied by fatigue, sleep, memory and mood issues."[14] It's a condition that affects 20 times more women than men, and it's greatly exacerbated by stress.

---

11 Shallenberger. Peripheral neuropathy cured in seven days: 3.
12 Rowen R. *Second Opinion.* 2007;17(7).
13 Fuchs N. Proven ways to relieve the terrible pain of shingles. *Women's Health Letter.* March 2002.
14 Definition of Fibromyalgia. http://www.mayoclinic.com/health/fibromyalgia/DS00079 Accessed August 16, 2013.

One of the physicians who have done pioneering work in the treatment of fibromyalgia is Jorge Flechas, M.D. He notes that for a long time doctors thought this condition was psychosomatic – that it was all in the patient's head. "In medicine, a lot of times a 'disease' does not exist until we find a drug for it, but once we have a drug approved by the FDA made by some pharmaceutical company, then all of a sudden the disease 'exists.'"[15] So, in the absence of any treatment protocol, he began questioning his patients to find what kind of things relieved the pain for them. He found that orgasm caused relief from the pain for three to four hours. Similarly, nursing a baby also caused relief from the pain.

What these things have in common is that they cause the body to release the hormone oxytocin. Orgasm, for instance, causes body levels of oxytocin to increase by 365 percent.[16] This hormone is something of an anti-stress hormone, and it tends to relieve the pain associated with fibromyalgia accordingly.

He began treating a few of his patients with an intravenous solution of saline and oxytocin. This treatment proved successful, but the IV benefits lasted for only 18 hours. Continued IV use was impractical, so he came up with oxytocin in pill form. It's a special form of pill needed because taking oxytocin orally allows it to be metabolized by the liver. The oxytocin never makes it to the rest of the body. These tablets embed oxytocin in a wax matrix, which prevents the liver from metabolizing it and allows it to be absorbed and distributed by the lymphatic system. This method of delivery has been clinically shown to increase levels of oxytocin in the blood within one hour.[17] These tablets must be made in a compounding pharmacy, so contact Dr. Flechas' office (see Resources section for contact info) for more information if this therapy is something you want to try.

There are some foods that increase oxytocin in the body, such as turkey, cottage cheese, nuts, fish, chicken, cheese, and eggs.[18] Whether these foods will give you enough of an oxytocin boost to help your fibromyalgia is a question you'll have to experiment with to determine. You may not match the extreme increase the body can provide, but you may find a combination of foods that gives you some relief.

Fibromyalgia sufferers typically suffer from cold hands and feet. This is because they are hypoxic (have poor oxygen) because of poor circulation, which is likely a major cause of the condition itself. Oxytocin works by opening up the capillaries and allowing a strong increase in circulation. This is the characteristic at work in the warm flush experienced after orgasm. It decreases stress, increases the sense of well-being, and greatly increases circulation. All of these

15   Burnett K, interview of Flechas J. The Potential of Oxytocin, Nitric Oxide, and Iodine. *Alternative Therapies.* 2013;19(4):51.

16   YouTube video: Oxytocin in Private Practice – Jorge D. Flechas, MD. http://www.youtube.com/watch?v=Y2mH O6QrKV0&feature=related. Accessed August 16, 2013.

17   Shallenberger F, interview of Flechas J. New breakthrough therapy stops fibromyalgia and increases female libido. *Real Cures.* 2010;9(8):6.

18   What foods contain oxytocin? http://www.ask.com/question/what-foods-contain-oxytocin. Accessed October 10, 2013.

effects combat fibromyalgia.

There are some very helpful dietary options to help increase circulation, as well. Both nattokinase and lumbrokinase are dietary supplements that are powerful clot and fibrin dissolvers (fibrin is a precursor of blood clots). Nattokinase is a traditional Japanese food made from fermented soybeans. Eating it is one of the most helpful things you can do for your circulatory health, as long as you can stand the taste. Finding it is not easy, however, so it has been put into capsules (which also solves the taste problem) and is available from many dietary supplement companies.

Lumbrokinase is made from earthworms. Like nattokinase, it's very helpful in boosting circulation and dissolving clots and fibrin deposits. Both products are available from the Allergy Research Group, allergyresearchgroup.com, 1-800-545-9960, and several other supplement companies online.

And finally – and surprisingly – temporomandibular joint disorders (TMJ) have a connection to fibromyalgia. Having a knowledgeable dentist or doctor address problems in the jaw or throat area often results in relief from fibromyalgia. You can read more on this subject in Chapter 20.

Chapter 6

Headache Pain

Most of us know headaches as an occasional nuisance, but they can be a very serious source of pain and disability. Regardless of how they manifest themselves to you, there are ways to treat them.

If your headache is one that causes dizziness and lightheadedness, your diet might be at fault. Hypoglycemia and insulin resistance can be caused by an excess of simple carbs such as sugars or bleached flour products. Cutting back on these, along with processed foods (which contain many simple carbs) and caffeine (which can overstimulate the adrenal gland and add to a hypoglycemic state) will often yield fast results. Keep these food items to a minimum – or cut them out entirely – and you will prevent this type of headache in the future.

Several essential oils can be used to obtain relief from mild to moderate headaches (see Chapter 9). Lavender is often used. It can be mixed with a carrier oil (three or four drops of lavender to a teaspoon to a tablespoon of olive oil, for instance). Wet a cotton ball with the mixture and dab it on your temples. You can also put a few drops of lavender oil into three cups of boiling water in a pan. Lean over the pan, drape a towel over your head and the pan, and breathe the concentrated vapors. Or you can put a few drops in a bath and soak in it.

DMSO can also be effective in relieving headache pain (also in Chapter 9). DMSO is a very potent substance that is effective in relieving a number of kinds of pain. It is cheap, readily available, and highly therapeutic in healing soft tissue injuries (muscle tears, sprains, etc.) You can just massage it into the scalp or temples over the site of the headache pain for what can often be quick and thorough relief.

You'll read in Chapter 10 that a woman suffered horrible headaches for 16 years before the source of the problem was identified. She had an infected tooth, which was quickly and completely remedied by the use of a Class III medical laser in a treatment called low level laser therapy (LLLT). Once the bacteria beneath the tooth were killed, her headaches went away and stayed away.

If your headaches are caused by anything related to an oxygen deficiency (indicated by shortness of breath, distress at altitude – such as in high mountains or on a plane, being rapidly winded by activity) or a condition that is helped by supplemental oxygen therapies, a number of the treatments in Chapter 12 might be helpful. Specifically, intravenous hydrogen peroxide therapy, hyperbaric oxygen therapy, and exercise with oxygen therapy can be helpful.

And a number of the manipulative therapies can also be helpful for headaches. Depending on the reason for the headache, osteopathic or chiropractic manipulation can often be of help. This is particularly true if the problem is in the cervical vertebrae (those in the upper part of the spinal column, just below the skull). If the problem is tension-related, a massage therapist can be of immense help. And zero balancing and craniosacral therapy are almost tailor-made for headache relief. These techniques often get to the cause of the headache, which prevents the problem from coming back in the future. See Chapter 14 for more information.

Section 3

The Wide, Wide World of Treatment Options Available Today

You'll see in this section a truly wide array of treatment options. Some you'll probably have heard a great deal about, such as exercise and nutrition. I've tried to put these subjects in something of a new and thoughtful form so you won't be tempted to view them as "been there, done that." Though they are often discussed in every imaginable forum, the plain fact is that they are astoundingly powerful therapeutic modalities. Any person wanting to relieve their pain ignores them at their peril.

Other therapies here will probably be new to you. My hope is that you will not only find something of interest, but something of use. I have therefore offered some of the most powerful and wide-ranging pain therapies available.

Part 1

The Basics

In just about every field, success comes down to the basics. In health, the basics are nutrition and exercise. Get them right and everything else becomes easier. Get them wrong and you're constantly fighting uphill. Volumes have been written about both nutrition and exercise, but in the following pages you'll find what you need to know about them as they relate to pain.

Topical treatments might be a step beyond the basics, but the step is not a big one. Even kids know to rub a sore spot. Throw in an essential oil or some DMSO and you've got a great way to treat many sources of pain. The treatments we'll discuss in the last chapter of this part are derived from plants or wood – still pretty low on the complexity scale.

Chapter 7

Eat to Ease Your Pain

Let's turn our attention now to the things you can do about the various kinds of pain you might be dealing with. Nutrition is first. It's not new, but it's the single most important thing you can do for your health. If you're of a conventional turn of mind, medically speaking, that will seem like an incredible claim. If you've studied the matter, it will seem elementary. Nonetheless, it is simply true. Everything you want to do to improve your health or relieve your pain will be made more effective through good nutrition – often dramatically so. Often astoundingly so.

I'm an old meat-and-potatoes kind of guy, so my making the above statement represents a pilgrimage of the intellect that has taken several years and a very gradual rewiring of my mind on the subject. I grew up eating whatever struck my fancy, and I thought it was my duty as a red-blooded American male to eat lots of processed foods and lots of simple carbs. It's been in only the last 20 years or so that I've seen how counterproductive that is to both my health and the way I feel on a daily basis.

Eating right promotes health, helps heal disease and injury, and can help you think and feel better. More pertinent to the topic at hand, proper nutrition can substantially decrease joint and muscle pain, as well as some kinds of skin pain. Some kinds of headache pain can also be dealt with nutritionally, as can many digestive problems. (Whether the latter can accurately be described as painful probably depends on the individual, but they are certainly uncomfortable.)

Which is not to say all of the nutritional advice out there is worth taking, or even healthy. Much of it is geared toward weight loss, and can actually help with that goal for a period of time, but can also detract from your health by depriving you of needed nutrients or balance in your diet. Diets modeled on populations that have maintained good health for long periods of time can be extremely healthful and efficacious in both the short and long term, such as the Mediterranean Diet or certain Asian diets – particularly the Japanese. (A few books describing such diets are listed in the Resources section.) But if you engage in crash diets or fad diets such as eating nothing but bananas for a month, I can almost guarantee that both your weight and your health will decrease. And when you resume your normal diet, the weight will return – your health, perhaps more slowly, if at all (depending on what your "normal" diet is).

One of the best diets proposed in recent years was first billed as the "no-grain diet." Later, to satisfy the college-educated urban/suburban folks[19] who buy most of the diet books, it was billed as the Paleolithic diet, or the caveman diet. It reflects the diet of hunter-gatherer tribes

---

19   Nothing derogatory here – I've got a few college degrees and I've lived in the suburbs – just a factual description of the audience for most of the diet books.

supposedly living in the long-ago past, modeled on a theory of human origins popular with the target audience. The truth is that hunter-gatherers have existed at all time periods of human existence, and they exist by the hundreds of thousands, if not millions, today. If their diet was everything its advocates say it is, Yanomamo tribesman – who have immediate and unfettered access to all the treasures of the rainforest – would have a lock on all the medals at every four-year Olympic competition. As a Maquiritare tribesman from Venezuela once told a fawning American anthropologist: "If you think tromping through the jungle all day trying to catch something to eat while getting eaten alive by vampire gnats is so wonderful, go right ahead."[20]

The caveman diet is healthful not because of any predisposition in human biology for the fare supposedly eaten by a romanticized version of hunter-gatherers, but because unprocessed, basic foods from naturally grown sources have more of the nutrients in them that people need and less of the toxins that harm their health. This is not rocket science. If you put good gas in your car, it runs better. If you put good food in your stomach, you run better. What the diet proponents are basically advising people to do is to buck the economic system that produces mediocre, industrialized fare at low cost for hundreds of millions of people. That's good advice, but, not surprisingly, bucking that system can be expensive – hence the diet's primary market is sophisticated, well-heeled city folk who are simultaneously inclined to buy into health trends and affluent enough to afford the foods the diet requires.

To eat well on a budget, you can still abide by many of the guidelines of this way of eating. You might not be able to constantly buy or grow organic foods (which, though an excellent and important thing to do, is also quite expensive), but you can omit many of the most harmful items. Your diet will be known almost as well for what it cuts out as for what it includes. And there's a definite monetary benefit: *Not* eating a food is cheap!

First, cut out sugar and all its alternatives and substitutes, except perhaps stevia, xylitol, or luoganhuo. Sugar is not a grain, but it is the most serious dietary threat to your health, no exaggeration (along with its most common substitute today: high fructose corn syrup). When you eat sugar, it is absorbed into your blood through your intestinal wall. Too much blood sugar is bad for your circulation, eyes, kidneys, and just about everything else. It can reduce the blood flow to your capillaries, which are your smallest blood vessels. High blood sugar causes your pancreas to secrete insulin, which is your body's natural counterbalance to sugar, and regulates how much of it is available to bodily tissues.

If you constantly consume sugar, the amount of insulin produced by your body to control it eventually becomes a problem. Insulin converts excess sugar into fat, with all the problems that entails. Excessive insulin has even been identified as a risk factor for prostate cancer.[21] More commonly, you'll develop what's called insulin resistance, in which your bodily tissues no longer

---

20   Bomer M. The anthropologists' "paradise." *World.* 1996;11(27).
21   Hammarsten J, Högstedt B. Hyperinsulinemia: a prospective risk factor for lethal clinical prostate cancer." *Eur J Cancer.* 2005;41(18):2887-95.

react properly to the insulin produced. When that happens, you start having problems controlling your blood sugar, and you run the risk of developing diabetes. Not only will wounds or injuries heal slowly in the presence of this condition, many will not heal at all. Diabetes, where blood-sugar control is virtually lost, can cause cardiovascular disease (sometimes even necessitating amputation of limbs due to complications related to poor blood circulation), kidney failure, and retinal (eye) disease. Weight gain and overall poor health are common characteristics of the condition.

For the same reason that you should cut out sugar, cut out all simple carbohydrates. Simple carbohydrates are so called because they have simple molecular structures that are very easily broken down in the human digestive system. They also have high levels of dietary sugars, which, like table sugar and other sugars, spike insulin levels quickly and flood the body with high levels of that hormone. For both these reasons, eating a piece of white bread has much the same effect on the body as eating a piece of candy.

Wheat flour, especially the bleached variety, is one of the worst offenders in this category. Fruit juice, cake, jam, biscuits, molasses, soda, and packaged cereals are also problematic. Most grains are also serious offenders – hence the rationale for the no-grain diet. But while a diet that issues a blanket prohibition on grains is easy to abide by because it is easily understood, it's not necessarily optimal advice. Some grains (or grain-like seeds), such as oats, flax, and quinoa, are extremely healthy, and need not be avoided. But if you're an all-or-nothing kind of person, as many of us can be at times, by all means go grain-free. The advantages will far outweigh the disadvantages. Among other benefits, it will keep you away from virtually all processed foods, almost all of which contain grains or sugar (and many other unhealthy ingredients).

This advice alone is often enough to control arthritis pain. Diet has been clinically demonstrated to help rheumatoid arthritis,[22] but few such studies have been conducted. Why is that? Because treating arthritis with drugs is big business, so the incentive to treat it with diet is limited to alternative practitioners and individuals – who have little means to conduct trials on the subject. Anecdotal evidence is far more plentiful. If you are not impressed with such evidence, you might have a problem with where I'm going at this point. But you can settle the matter quickly and easily by simply trying it yourself. If you suffer from arthritis, stop eating sugars and grains for a month. Most such foods are empty calories, so you risk nothing, health-wise, by doing so. You'll see for yourself that your health will gain a great deal from doing this – whether or not it significantly helps your arthritis.

I have early-stage arthritis in the knuckles on both hands. It is easily controlled in precisely this manner. If I engage in a chocoholic binge, my fingers suffer intense pain the next day. If I lay off the sugar and baked goods, the pain goes away. It's not science, but neither is my habit of flicking on the switch near the door each time I enter a room. Almost invariably, a light in the

22 Darlington L, Ramsey NW, and Mansfield JR. Placebo controlled, blind study of dietary manipulation therapy in rheumatoid arthritis, *Lancet.* 1986;327(8475):236-238.

room comes on, though this relationship between switch and light has not been scientifically proven in a randomized, double-blind, placebo-controlled clinical trial.

This underscores what I emphasized earlier about the need for you to *think*. Modern medical research is an important contribution to scientific inquiry and the search for truth, but biased or dishonest researchers can easily undermine it. In the United States, it is largely used to support the medical-industrial complex, in which high-cost solutions that line the pockets of vested medical interests are almost invariably favored over simple, low-cost, natural alternatives. It is very common for trial outcomes to favor the products or procedures of those who pay for them (this can be as true for alternative therapies as conventional ones). The structure of the trial or the interpretation of it can be subtly altered to obtain the desired outcome.

A second point to make in this regard is that the scientific method has limits. It is complex, time-consuming, resource-intensive, and therefore very expensive. It consequently favors matters in which substantial financial interests are at stake, despite the fact that it is most useful to the population at large when it is used to discover low-cost solutions for serious health problems. Said bluntly: If what is being tested is not lucrative, few can afford to test it. Exceptions to this way of doing things are fortunately becoming more common, but it definitely describes the dominant force in "scientific" testing.

A third important point is that truth can be determined in many ways. Most of what you know to be true in life was not revealed to you as such by the scientific method. You didn't learn to walk because a clinical trial revealed that putting one foot in front of the other was the best way for humans to propel themselves to where they want to go. Nor did you need a study to tell you that putting your hand on a hot stovetop was detrimental to your well-being. The scientific method consists of organizing and conducting many anecdotes in a restricted manner that allows them to be meaningfully analyzed. As such, in an important sense, it is anecdotal medicine, as well (which is not to minimize its potential for determining complex truths, *if properly conducted*).

You can often achieve some of the same results by thoughtfully conducting and carefully analyzing many anecdotes of your own, using yourself as a subject. I would strongly encourage you to do so, with the important caveat that you thoroughly understand and weigh the risks involved before doing so. In the case of diet, and especially in the case of limiting your simple-carb intake, the risk is effectively zero, even as the upside is quite large.

Many people are frightened away from alternative medicine because of a lack of clinical trial support for any given modality. The above discussion should go far toward explaining why this is so often the case. Tens of thousands, perhaps hundreds of thousands, of people have sharply reduced the pain from, if not cured, their arthritis using diet. Yet conventional medicine advocates point to a lack of scientific proof for this approach. They have a uniquely effective way of pouring disdain on anything that competes with them for patient loyalty, and thus, in their case, patient dollars.

If you doubt this, look up some of the treatments mentioned in this report on wikipedia.org. Most of the medical entries on that site are written by conventional health practitioners, and either damn the procedure with faint praise or cast doubt on it with snooty, condescending references to the lack of science supporting its efficacy.

Be very careful when reading or listening to such analysis. It is far from objective, though it masquerades as the most objective evaluation possible – hiding behind the rubric of "science." Most of the treatments in this report are characterized by two things: A very significant upside for those for whom a given treatment works, and a very minimal – often nonexistent – downside for everyone who tries it. A significant number also offer low cost. With characteristics like that, the decision ought to be easy. But it can be complicated by "experts" who make it seem foolish or irresponsible to try anything not in the mainstream of their exceptionally costly brand of medicine.

Basic Nutrition

Having established what's important to cut out of your diet, I don't want to minimize what's important for good nutrition. The organic market has quickly established itself as a high-cost, if very healthy, alternative to industrial fare. That's reflective of the economic realities involved in producing foods without modern insecticides, pesticides, and breeding or genetic modification that maximizes production advantages rather than taste or nutrition. But even if organic food's expense is economically defensible for producers, it can be brutal to families on a budget.

Good nutrition is expensive – either in money or in time and effort. But recent advances in things like aquaponics (the growing of mutually nourishing vegetable- and fish-producing systems in a greenhouse), composting, mulching, and natural insecticides have given home growers a way to live healthy without breaking the bank. See the Resources section for some great insights into these advances. Some of the work being done in these fields is truly amazing.

And if growing your own food or buying organic isn't possible (though you can do some of it in an apartment under a window or on a balcony), be sure to augment your diet with nutritional supplements. A full exposition of optimal human nutrition is beyond the scope of this report, but nutritional deficiencies are the cause of many kinds of pain. Magnesium deficiencies can cause muscle cramps and spasms, along with much more serious conditions; vitamin C deficiency can slow the healing of your wounds; vitamin D deficiency can cause rickets in children or osteoporosis (bone loss) in adults. And the list goes on quite extensively. Few wounds, diseases, or injuries can heal well without good nutrition.

Common multivitamins seldom offer enough of any given nutrient to make much difference, but many physician-directed supplement makers now offer vitamin and nutrient products that are of high quality and sufficient quantity to make a genuine difference in health. Again, see the Resources section for information on these products.

Anti-Inflammation Foods

Chronic inflammation is such a huge problem, and such a serious contributor to chronic pain, that it might behoove you to look into its dietary solutions on a more item-by-item basis. Using a no-grain diet or a Mediterranean or Japanese diet will likely work for you, but variety remains the spice of life – and people also vary in their reaction to foods.

Some key foods you'll want to know about include curcumin (from the spice turmeric); omega-3-rich foods such as flax and cold-water fish (and their oils, which are available as supplements at the health-food store); nuts; vitamin K2 (found in natto; fermented vegetables; and brie, gouda, and edam cheeses); fruits such as blueberries, cranberries, and cherries; cruciferous vegetables such as broccoli and cauliflower; cocoa; ginger; nettle leaf; ginkgo biloba; bromelain; and grass-fed beef. These foods strongly counteract chronic inflammation.

A study published in *Gut*[23] found that the curry pigment curcumin not only reduced inflammation, but reduced liver cell damage and scarring. This might make curcumin good for those with hepatitis or damage from alcohol, chemicals, or drugs. Those who have treated their serious chronic pain with liver-damaging drugs might well enjoy a significant double benefit from this potent nutrient. To get enough of it without losing all your friends (curry's effect on a person's … aroma … is similar to that of garlic), you'll probably want to take a concentrated dose in a supplement. One possibility is Curamed, which comes in 500 mg capsules – one capsule, three times a day.

Another study looked at the nutritional benefit of nuts.[24] This food is a rich source of alpha-linolenic acid, which is a plant-derived omega-3 fatty acid. Omega-3 has long been recognized as a potent anti-inflammatory nutrient. The study, however, showed that nuts were a superior source of protection from death (up to a 51% reduction in death from inflammatory disease among those who ate the most nuts) to fish oil. While no mention was made in the study regarding pain reduction from eating nuts, such reduction is common from fish oil. I would certainly recommend trying nuts in this regard. They are a healthful and delicious way to experiment.

A family of foods you might try eliminating if your inflammation persists after eliminating grains and sugar might be the nightshades. Many people have allergies to these foods, and these allergies can trigger a white blood cell response that in turn causes inflammation. Nightshades include potatoes, tomatoes, peppers, eggplants, and some spices. It's easy to develop an addiction to these foods, which makes them very hard to give up. And potato starch, for instance, can be found in many frozen and processed foods, so potato starch from these sources can be hard to eliminate from your diet. But doing so might be just the thing that relieves your arthritis pain.

23   Baghdasaryan A, Claudell T, Kosters A, et al. Curcumin improves sclerosing cholangitis in Mdr2$^{-/-}$ mice by inhibition of cholangiocyte inflammatory response and portal myofibroblast proliferation. *Gut.* 2010;59:521-530. doi:10.1136/gut.2009.186528

24   Gopinath B, Buyken AE, Flood VM, Empson M, Rochtchina E, Mitchell P. Consumption of polyunsaturated fatty acids, fish, and nuts and risk of inflammatory disease mortality. *Am J Clin Nutr.* 2011;93(5).

Nan Kathryn Fuchs, Ph.D., had one patient who tried every arthritis treatment she could find, but experienced no success until she did away with her daily glass of tomato juice – which alleviated her arthritis entirely. It's worth trying.[25]

In recent years, researchers have looked at the inflammatory nature of many foods, even producing books with extensive tables and documentation. One such book is *The Inflammation Free Diet Plan*, by Monica Reinagel. The author extensively tested literally hundreds of foods to determine their "IF" ratings (IF being "inflammation free"), and these ratings are published in the book. Each food has either a positive or negative numerical rating that indicates how inflammatory it is. A food with a rating of 493, such as grilled wild Atlantic salmon, is highly inflammation-free, or non-inflammatory. But a food with a rating of -202, such as a serving of Rice Krispies, is a strongly inflammatory food to put in your stomach.

Ms. Reinagel's was one of the earlier and more exhaustive efforts to catalogue foods by their inflammatory tendencies in the human body. Entire meal plans are recommended based on IF ratings. If you suffer from inflammation-related pain, and want more variety than the no-grain diet offers, I would definitely recommend trying some or many of these meals. While I cannot attest to the accuracy of Ms. Reinagel's numbers, her methodology and the gist of her research appear sound. At a minimum, her method provides a useful framework on which to evaluate foods. Testing her theory is an exercise in eating wholesome foods in researched combinations. That's an evaluation most people would find somewhat less than objectionable, and probably quite enjoyable.

---

25   Fuchs NC. Beyond a healthy diet — eliminate nightshades. *Women's Health Letter*, October 2003.

Chapter 8

Get Up and Do Something

You're doubtless tired of hearing "eat right and exercise" as the solution to all health problems, or at least the way to prevent them. The advice is too simple – and too hard. For many it's not much fun, and for many others it's purest drudgery. Those objections can largely be addressed, but in this case the popular mantra is absolutely correct. And it's correct to a far greater degree than many people ever realize.

There are a number of ways exercise is important to pain prevention or relief. By helping with weight control, it keeps excess strain off of joints. Such strain can be a major contributor to joint pain. (Diet can also relieve strain on joints by way of reducing weight.)

By increasing blood flow, exercise provides more blood supply to the joints, which normally experience far less blood (and thus oxygen) presence than most other bodily tissues. Even if arthritis prevents very much exercise at all, it's important to move the joints if possible. If you don't, virtually all movement will eventually become too painful.

Although joint tissues such as ligaments, tendons, and cartilage do not respond to exercise as muscles do, they are nourished by the additional blood flow and kept supple and vital by movement and subtle strain. When these tissues are strong and uninjured, they keep joints moving in the right range of movement. This prevents injury to the joint, and also prevents pain from improper motion – either acute or chronic.

One type of exercise that is seldom given its due except by its more extreme practitioners is resistance exercise such as weight lifting or bodyweight exercises – or even exercising in water for mild resistance appropriate to those recuperating from serious injuries or starting out from an extreme out-of-condition state. You needn't be a weight lifting competitor or body builder to benefit from it. Indeed, it is one of the most helpful things you can do for yourself, no matter your age or physical condition.

The *New England Journal of Medicine* published a study of exercise done with people over 70 years of age.[26] Almost 40 percent of the subjects were in their 90s; 83 percent required a cane, walker, or wheelchair at the beginning of the study; two thirds of them had fallen in the past year; 50 percent had arthritis; 44 percent had pulmonary disease; 44 percent had osteoporotic fracture; 35 percent had hypertension; and 24 percent had cancer. This was not a study of athletes in the prime of life.

---

26 Fiatarone MA, O'Neill EF, Ryan ND, et al. Exercise training and nutritional supplementation for physical frailty in very elderly people. *N Engl J Med.* 1994;330;1769-1775.

The study lasted 10 weeks, and followed 63 women and 37 men. Only the hip and knee extensors were trained in the study, which was done with gym equipment (though it can be done at home, as well). Each participant determined the maximum weight he or she could lift in each exercise, and trained with 80 percent of that weight. As they were able, this weight was increased. They trained three days a week for 45 minutes per session, with at least a day in between each training day. They did three sets of eight repetitions of each lift, with each repetition lasting six to nine seconds, with one to two seconds between reps and two minutes of rest between sets.

For those (over 90 percent) who finished the study, the results were that average muscle strength increased by 113 percent, walking speed increased by 11.8 percent, power for climbing stairs increased by 28.4 percent, and thigh muscle size (determined cross-sectionally) increased by 2.7 percent. They could walk farther and were more stable on their feet. Over 35 percent of those who were confined to chairs before the study were subsequently able to not only walk, but climb stairs.

Clearly, resistance exercise is a huge functionality enhancer, but how about pain relief? A study was published in the *Journal of Strength & Conditioning Research* that looked at pain perception before, during, and after conducting resistance training.[27] The study was specifically intended to see if there was a difference in perception that depended on when the exercise was done, whether in the morning or the evening. It found that time was not a factor, but that resistance exercise significantly reduced perceived pain after as little as one minute.

Much more importantly, the benefits last beyond the exercise period. Danish scientists at the National Research Center for the Working Environment in Copenhagen found that women who did five neck muscle-strengthening exercises consistently over time found long-lasting relief from their pain.[28] Since neck pain from sitting at a computer all day is one of the fastest growing complaints of our time, this is particularly good news (though the study findings are doubtless extensible to other kinds of pain, particularly those derived from poor posture or repetitive motion). The exercises are described and pictured at an easily accessible online page from Harvard Medical School.[29]

Benefits to the muscles and cardiovascular system from exercise have been so voluminously dealt with in every possible medium that I won't go into them at length here. One benefit from exercise-induced muscular development that isn't always mentioned, however, is that it can help stabilize joints that suffer from injured or stretched ligaments. Muscles are quite inferior to ligaments in this role, but they are far from useless. Doing appropriate exercises to strengthen the muscles attached to the joint can help prevent further injury to a knee, for instance,

27   Focht BC; Koltyn KF. Alterations in pain perception after resistance exercise performed in the morning and evening. *J Strength & Conditioning Research*. 2009;23(3):891-897. doi: 10.1519/JSC.0b013e3181a05564
28   Andersen LL, Kjær M, Søgaard K, Hansen L, Kryger AI, Sjøgaard G. Effect of two contrasting types of physical exercise on chronic neck muscle pain. *Arthritis Care & Research*. 2008;59(1):84-91.
29   Strength training resolves chronic neck pain. HEALTHbeat. www.health.harvard.edu/healthbeat/HEALTH-beat_042908.htm. Accessed August 20, 2013.

though they will not restore full strength or rigor to the joint.

The body must move as it was intended (or as closely as possible to that ideal) if it is to move well and avoid pain. Imagine a Swiss watch, with its myriad gears, levers, and springs. If something gets out of place or some dust gets in the gears, it will not keep good time. It might even stop. Every component has a proper axis on which to turn, a proper range within which to work, or a specific pressure to exert. Violate the parameters within which it was intended to work, and it won't – work, that is.

Your body is far, far more complex than a Swiss watch, and its parameters of operation are sometimes more flexible, but the principle is the same. Extend a limb beyond its operational limits, and you'll injure the ligaments that keep the pivotal joint stable.

When a football player from Columbia University thought that spearing my left knee with his head was a good way to keep me from blocking a punt (it was), I became acquainted with this fact. My kneecap ripped loose and was pushed to the left side of my knee, and my leg bent backward by tens of degrees farther than it was supposed to go. It gave me a short-term introduction to the long-term severe pain some people endure, and it ended my football career – such as it was. Far more seriously, it altered the physiology of my knee.

Fortunately, I was still able to function and complete a great deal of rigorous military training. But during all of that often-brutal training, my left knee was always my weak link. Even now, it allows me to easily hyperextend my leg. This can cause a jarring effect when I walk if I don't concentrate on keeping it bent just a little bit at its furthest extension. I'm not able to do that if I don't keep the muscles of my leg in shape. The ligaments and tendons allow me to extend my leg too far, but my muscles can prevent that problem – if they're in shape. So I'm highly dependent on exercise for my continued mobility.

If you have a similar joint injury (and the ligaments aren't severed – only surgery can address severed ligaments), first seriously consider prolozone (Chapter 13), PEMF (Chapter 11), or FSM (Chapter 21) treatments (unfortunately, these weren't available when I injured my knee). Getting these treatments early can make a *huge* difference in how quickly and thoroughly your injury heals.

But second, be sure to exercise as much as is appropriate for the injury. To determine what's appropriate for a significant injury, you may need a professional opinion if you don't have a good knowledge of human biology or exercise physiology (which, with a little diligence and an Internet connection you can easily acquire these days). If you'd prefer not to visit a doctor or chiropractor, an exercise trainer will often work wonders in this regard. The latter are trained to teach you exercises that will support and restore normal function to your injured limb or joint – and they can be very helpful in this capacity. If you opt to go it alone, however, do some research, and remember the "don't do that!" precept. If it hurts…

Because I was not aware of any of these therapies when I was injured, exercise has been by far the most helpful thing I've done to maintain the use of my knee. And listen, I'm trying to strike a fine balance here between trying several do-it-yourself options and getting medical help. Either option can be frustrating, I know. I've done them both. Doctors are expensive and often do the wrong thing (for which they charge the same as for doing the right thing – often more). And doing it yourself often entails many false starts and lots of time, energy, and even money.

Once you've educated yourself about some basic physiology and some of the options that can be helpful in situations like yours, sometimes the best thing is to just sit back and think. What's the problem? What seems like it would help? You'll probably come up with a theory or two. Assess the risks. If the reward/risk ratio is highly favorable, give it a try (*very* gently, at first). If it seems to help, do more of it. If it hurts, put that information into the gray matter and try another tack. Some of my best solutions are combinations of what I've read or been told or shown and what I've done to improve the technique for my personal situation. So take charge of your situation and do whatever it takes to make things better.

Here are a few suggestions to get you started:

- If you can do so without significant distortion of your normal gait due to pain or injury, walking is almost always a very good thing to do. It's easy, healthful, and enjoyable. Just be sure you have some comfortable shoes and a safe route to walk (not just safe from muggers; safe from rocks, cracked pavement, and uneven ground; I have turned an ankle several times on such minor things). Not much else is required.

- Biking is also excellent. It's great cardiovascular exercise, and it moves your back, hips, knees, and ankles through a significant range of motion without applying any injurious out-of-axis or out-of-range forces to them. In essence, your joints are virtually locked into a very healthy range of motion. If your place of residence doesn't offer good biking opportunities, bike indoors. You can either use a stationary bicycle or a regular bike on an indoor trainer. To train indoors, even a single speed bike is fine. Some trainers have variable resistance features. If you're not familiar with bike trainers, go to amazon.com and type in "bike resistance trainer" to see what I'm referring to. It's basically a steel stand that attaches to your back axle and lifts and applies resistance to the rear tire as you pedal. If you don't want to buy new, you can go to craigslist.com or ebay.com and pick up both a bicycle and trainer for much less than retail.

- Kettlebells are an excellent way to get in some resistance exercises. If you're not familiar with them, again check out amazon.com. Just type in "kettlebell" and you'll see what they are. They look like cast-iron bowling balls with big fat handles on them. Youtube.com offers a number of videos that can acquaint you with how they're used. They're excellent for your joints because, unlike barbells, they do not require you to lift the weight with your joints in a fixed position. Each joint is able to seek out its best position, which stresses it far less than either traditional free weights (except dumbbells) or machine weights.

- Kettlebells are a bit of a fad right now, which means that, new, they are very expensive. However, as with most fads, they lose their luster for many people very quickly. (Unlike many fads, they really work. They were first used extensively by Russian Special Forces, and they're very effective.) You can therefore sometimes pick them up on craigslist or at garage sales for a song. I recommend the lacquered or painted cast iron bells rather than those covered with vinyl. The vinyl looks nice, but it pulls the hair on your arm as you're lifting. Not a serious problem, but a distraction, at least.

- If you're a capable swimmer, swimming is one of the best exercises you can do. It's basically a combination of resistance and cardiovascular training, and gives you benefits common to each of those categories of exercise. If you're not a good swimmer, you can still do some cardio exercises while standing in water ranging from hip-deep to neck-deep. Many of the exercises demonstrated on TV or on youtube.com for cardiovascular training can be done in the water, to even greater effect and with significantly less risk (if you lose your balance and fall, it's no big deal because water cushions your fall).

- Jogging is not a good exercise for your joints (I say this both as someone who has jogged thousands of miles and because of researchers who have come to the same conclusion). Particularly as you get older, the stress it puts on mid- and lower-body joints and the wear it causes joint cartilage can be significant. Biking, cross-country skiing, walking, and swimming are far easier on the joints, while still offering significant cardiovascular benefits.

- If you're not sure where to start, join a gym or recreation center with good exercise facilities. Join one that doesn't require a long-term commitment, if possible. Your goal is to learn what you like best and what suits your needs best. If you prefer, you can exercise at home once you've learned that (if your preference doesn't involve lots of expensive equipment). Most gyms have knowledgeable staff that will help you learn exercises appropriate to your needs, no matter your level of experience. (I'm referring to exercise, not physical therapy. Don't expect them to know how to help you deal with or avoid aggravating an injury. A physical therapist, athletic trainer, chiropractor, or osteopath is necessary for that. A gym is where it's extremely important to remember the "if it hurts" rule. But for prevention, or to maintain optimum strength, flexibility, and balance, exercise can't be beat, and a good gym or recreation center is a great place to learn.)

- These days, some well-known organizations post excellent step-by-step exercise instructions online. I'm referring here to therapeutic exercises, such as for back pain. If you just type "back pain exercises" into your search engine, you'll instantly see Web sites for WebMD, the Cleveland Clinic, the Mayo Clinic, Prevention, and many sites by individual doctors who specialize in this area. Try some of these, remembering the "if it hurts…" rule. You can quickly put together a routine that gives you a good workout and also strengthens your body in a way that speeds healing and prevents further injury. To top it all off, the instruction is totally free, and many of the exercises require nothing more than a padded floor (such as a carpet or an exercise pad).

Chapter 9

Topical Treatments

Topical treatments can be surprising in their efficacy. It doesn't seem like they would have broad application given that many injuries occur far beneath the skin, but they can penetrate to a surprising depth, and they have mechanisms of action that are quite effective. Particularly for skin, subcutaneous (under the skin), and soft tissue pain or injuries, topical treatments can work well.

Essential oils

Essential oils are the oils taken from plants by expression (being squeezed out), distillation (being steamed out), or by using solvents (being leached out). They tend to retain many of the crucial substances present in each plant, thus representing its essence – hence an essential oil. They are much easier to store than the plants themselves, and they last longer and are easier to use, as well.

A given application of an oil will typically use only one to four drops, so although the oils seem expensive for the quantity you buy, they go a long way. And you need so little of them because they are extremely powerful. Simply applying many of them to the skin full strength will irritate the skin, so they are often mixed with another oil to dilute their strength. And for internal use, some users consider more than a drop of lavender, for instance, to a quart of water to be too much. These are truly powerful substances.

Plants often have remarkable medicinal applications, so having the essence of plants in an easily storable and usable oil is a significant advantage. To see what I mean regarding the usefulness of plants, perhaps a well-known product will be a good example. White willow bark has been well known as a pain reliever for centuries, if not millennia. Its active compound is salicin. Coincidentally (actually not), this is the active ingredient in aspirin. Aspirin, like many drugs in common use, was developed from known effective plant compounds. The compounds are typically purified, modified, concentrated, and standardized (and then often patented, to secure exclusive rights and large profit margins), but they are often very similar in characteristics to the plant compounds from which they were drawn. Today, you can get an essential oil from wintergreen that contains over 90 percent methyl salicylate. Not surprisingly, this oil is a good one to use for pain relief.

If you'd like to see what essential oils contain, and how many there are, you might find the Essential Oil University helpful, at essentialoils.org. It contains information on 2,571 oils and 3,260 compounds at this writing. It contains no narrative information on the oils, but lists in significant detail the compounds each contains, and what percentage of the total they represent. You'll have to register to gain access to this information, but this is not a commercial site. I've never been contacted for any purpose, marketing or otherwise, after registering.

Some essential oils can be taken internally, some are typically used for topical application or as massage oils in a mix with a carrier oil (such as olive oil), and some can be used aromatically, either directly or through a diffuser (a device to diffuse, or spread, the vaporized oil through the air in a room). With thousands of essential oils available, the subject is clearly a field all by itself, and can consume thousands of hours of study and application to become expert in the matter. Fortunately, that's not necessary. Many people have put in that time, and have written manuals or other study materials to help people new to the field find their way. A few of these are listed a little later in this chapter.

But you can know just a few things about essential oils and immediately begin to realize benefit from them. If you have Internet access, you might want to do a search for "essential oil toolkit." Several people have provided Web pages on this subject, and it's instructive to see what they consider the *essential* essential oils, so to speak. Lavender, peppermint, and tea tree (or melaleuca) seem to top many people's lists, with lemon a possible fourth gotta-have. These are for a wide variety of uses, however, not just for pain, so our focus on pain will diverge a bit from these.

Lavender, from the above list, does have significant pain-relieving capabilities. Massage Today confirms that, "Lavender is ... antimicrobial, anti-infectious, and antiseptic, making it effective in the treatment of wounds and as a frontline defense against respiratory infection.... Lavender is indicated for muscle spasm, sprain, strain, cramp, contracture, and rheumatic pain. It is sedative to the central nervous system and relieves headache, nervous tension, and insomnia...."[30]

Other useful oils are chamomile for headache, neuralgia, muscle and low back pain, and TMJ syndrome; clary sage as a massage oil to relieve spasm, muscle ache, and cramping; helichrysum for many of the same uses as lavender, as well as for bruising and burns; sweet marjoram, because of its highly sedative properties, for pain, stiffness, sprain, spasm, neuromuscular contractions, both rheumatoid and osteoarthritis, dysmenorrhea, and migraine; sandalwood for muscle spasm, sciatica, and lymph congestion; vetiver for arthritis, muscle ache, pain, sprain and stiffness, and to increase venous circulation to help detoxification of tissues.

These are all oils that should be used in a massage. A few drops (one to four, depending on the oil, is typical) of the essential oil is mixed with a teaspoon of carrier oil and the mix is then massaged into the skin. Some people believe that this method or inhaling the naturally occurring

---

30 Enteen S. Essential oils for pain relief. Massage Today. 2005;5(2). http://www.massagetoday.com/mpacms/mt/article.php?id=13161. Accessed September 6, 2013.

or diffused fumes are the best ways to get oils into the body. They bypass the stomach, with its destructive acid and enzymes, and go directly into the blood and tissues. Obviously this does not apply to oils used to aid digestion, but that's another subject.

If these uses and their results pique your interest in essential oils, I recommend buying a book with instructions and "recipes." The subject is vast, and more than I can responsibly cover in this report. Fortunately, several good books are available. *The Essential Oils Pocket Reference, 5th Edition*, May 2011 by Gary Young (2011), and *Modern Essentials: A Contemporary Guide to the Therapeutic Use of Essential Oils*, 4th Edition, by Aroma Tools (2012) are two books provided by essential oil products companies (*Pocket Reference* by Young Living, and *Modern Essentials* by doTerra). They cost between $22-24 new on Amazon.com. The upside of buying a book sponsored by a product company is that, as companies with liability for their products, the sponsors require the authors to list a good deal of safety information (e.g., conditions for which an oil is not recommended, ways not to use the oils). The downside is that the books are highly skewed to the products and proprietary blends offered by the companies. This is not necessarily bad, as both are good companies with good products, but it's something to be aware of.

Another book is *The Essential Oils Handbook: All the Oils You Will Ever Need for Health, Vitality and Well-Being* by Jennie Harding (2008). This is not an exhaustive reference book, as it is arranged practically by use rather than alphabetically by oil. But it's useful for a beginner or someone who intends limited use of oils on a practical basis (which includes the majority of essential oil users). (It's a small book with a small font, so don't get it if you have trouble reading small print.) It's less than $11 new on Amazon.com.

A short search online will often tell you how to use a specific oil for a specific purpose, and the cost of that is obviously free. You can find essential oils at your local health food store, or online. As mentioned above, Young Living and doTerra are two good brands, though both are multilevel marketing companies.[31] This adds to the cost, but the products are well regarded and have a good reputation for quality.

DMSO

Dimethylsulfoxide, or DMSO as it is commonly referred to, is one of the most widely useful substances you can have in your medicine cabinet. In its original use, it was an industrial solvent. But as you can see from the description below, it helps with a lot of things:

DMSO is used topically to decrease pain and speed the healing of wounds, burns, and muscle and skeletal injuries. DMSO is also used topically to treat painful conditions such

---

31   MLM is not a business model I like, even on a moral basis (I think it's a Ponzi scheme for distributors), but some MLM companies are easier to do business with than others. As with conventional medicine, I try to use the existing, much-bigger-than-I-am situation for my benefit. The better MLM companies put a good deal of research into new products and quite a bit of quality into all their products. You needn't shy away from them unless the price for their products is prohibitive or they require you to sell products for them to get their products.

as headache, inflammation, osteoarthritis, rheumatoid arthritis, and severe facial pain called tic douloureux. It is used topically for eye conditions including cataracts, glaucoma, and problems with the retina; for foot conditions including bunions, calluses, and fungus on toenails; and for skin conditions including keloid scars and scleroderma…. DMSO is used either alone or in combination with a drug called idoxuridine to treat pain associated with shingles (herpes zoster infection).[32]

Gabriela Segura, M.D., concisely describes some of its mechanism of action:

DMSO is an effective pain killer, blocking nerve conduction fibers that produce pain. It reduces inflammation and swelling by reducing inflammatory chemicals. It improves blood supply to an area of injury by dilating blood vessels and increasing delivery of oxygen and by reducing blood platelet stickiness. It stimulates healing, which is a key to its usefulness in any condition. It is among the most potent free radical scavengers known to man, if not the most potent one. This is a crucial mechanism since some molecules in our bodies produce an unequal number of electrons and the instability of the number causes them to destroy other cells. DMSO hooks on to those molecules and they are then expelled from the body with the DMSO.[33]

DMSO rapidly and easily penetrates the skin, so large quantities of it quickly reach deep tissues. It takes whatever is on the skin or on your hands with it, so make sure the area you're treating and your hands are clean – unless you have something, such as an essential oil solution, that you want to penetrate more deeply into your body.

In most cases, you can simply massage DMSO into the skin over the painful area. It's a safe treatment if used in this manner, but I recommend you bring a knowledgeable health practitioner into the picture if you want to treat eye problems or shingles.[34] It causes a smell like garlic to emanate from your skin, and you'll even taste it (a measure of how deeply and quickly it penetrates into the body). But if you can deal with the smell, the results are usually worth it.

DMSO can be an interesting exception to the "If it hurts…" rule. You can prove this to yourself (though I do *not* recommend it) by treating a sunburn with it. If you rub it on sunburned skin, there's a good chance you will heal and save the skin. However, the pain is excruciating. I do not tell you this theoretically.

---

32 Find a vitamin or supplement: DMSO (dimethylsulfoxide). WebMD. http://www.webmd.com/vitamins-supplements/ingredientmono-874-DMSO%20%28DIMETHYLSULFOXIDE%29.aspx?activeIngredientId=874&activeIngredientName=DMSO%20%28DIMETHYLSULFOXIDE%29. Accessed September 7, 2013.

33 Segura G. DMSO – the real miracle solution. Signs of the Times. http://www.sott.net/article/228453-DMSO-The-Real-Miracle-Solution. Accessed September 11, 2013.

34 Dr. Robert Rowen has developed a solution containing DMSO, glutathione, and vitamin C that helps about 40% of cataracts patients. Though he considers cataract surgery an excellent procedure, damage does sometimes occur. Thus, he recommends trying drops of this solution in the eyes before proceeding to surgery. His contact information is listed in the Resources section.

Bottom line on pain with DMSO: It's tricky. Try a little DMSO before you try a lot. It will probably sting. If it stings or hurts quite a bit, hold off for a while and see if there's any further adverse reaction. If there's not, you can start increasing the amount you use, knowing that the stinging is not indicative of a problem.

Athletes are especially aided by DMSO, as it is most useful for soft tissue injuries. Runners in particular used it extensively in the 1970s and 1980s.

"[DMSO] is most effective on soft tissue injuries, and generally speaking, the softer the better. For a stress fracture, don't waste your time. For tendonitis, ... it might help a little. Joint pain (a knee or ankle, especially if there is swelling) it's pretty effective. For a muscle pull or tear, it's pure money. In fact, in its 1980s heyday, it was primarily sprinters who raved about DMSO the most, since they were the most prone to muscle tears."[35]

DMSO is cheap and easily available at health food stores or online. It lasts a long time so it's a good idea to have some sitting in your medicine cabinet for many of the injuries life brings your way.

35   Hinkle C. DMSO: the best injury treatment you've never heard of. Dailymile. http://www.dailymile.com/blog/health/dmso-the-best-injury-treatment-youve-never-heard-of. Accessed September 7, 2013.

Part 2

Electromagnetic and Magnetic Therapies

This part of the report will cover one of the most exciting, powerful, and divisive fields of therapy you can name. Though electromagnetic radiation has many demonstrable physical effects on biological organisms, the suggestion that it can be therapeutic is panned outright by most conventional physicians. Nonetheless, as some uses continue to struggle to achieve wider acceptance, others have progressed to the stage of being FDA approved.

At present, many sources of therapeutic electromagnetic radiation are still prohibitively expensive for most people. Others, however, are extremely low-cost. Given that many of the more expensive machines are relatively simple electrical devices, they should come down in price as demand increases and manufacturing efficiencies are realized. Until then, some physicians make these therapies available at relatively low cost within their offices.

Chapter 10

Light Therapy

We come now to a subject that has the potential to divide the readership of this report rather sharply. To many people, light therapy belongs in a category with voodoo and witch doctors (of course some readers will find such a category intriguing). Such people might find something solid to stand on within the chapter on color therapy, where I try to put the medical applications of Eastern religion and Western scientism in some sort of perspective. Others have read material on it before, are acquainted with its science and claims, and are comfortable with it. Perhaps they have even tried and benefited from it.

Given the schism, let me try to ease people in the first category into this subject. Those in the second category can read ahead.

With any given category of treatment, perhaps it is useful to first establish that it can have an effect on human physiology – any effect, regardless of what it might be. Even if the effect is negative, at least the treatment can be seen to *do something*. It's not a big zero. From there, perhaps we can work our way to a logical postulate that something that affects organisms in a bad way can, when applied differently, have a good effect. After all, fire can burn people or it can warm them. Same element, same characteristics, different application, different outcome. Water or food can equally help or hurt.

Light is similar. We might think of it as helpful to see with, but of not much use beyond that. But life on earth could not exist without light – and that's not just because of the heat that accompanies it when we're talking about sunlight. Plants use sunlight to conduct photosynthesis – the converting of carbon dioxide (CO_2) and water (H_2O) into carbohydrates (consisting of carbon, hydrogen, and oxygen atoms, as the name suggests), which are important foods that nourish millions of life forms on earth. When subjected to pressure and heat, as when heavy forests are covered by flood deposition or the activity from a tectonic shift, these same atoms can form hydrocarbons (again, hydrogen and carbon) such as coal, oil, and natural gas, which power most of the machinery that keeps us safe, comfortable, and productive in modern society.

So light, in its most basic earthly application, is fundamental to human health. But that's an indirect application. We're going to talk about the direct application of light to the human body, so let's return to our negative-effect starting point. When you spend too much time in the sun without SPF-50 sun block or zinc oxide, what happens? You burn. If you do that too often, you may eventually find that sun damage can cause melanoma, a very serious and potentially fatal skin cancer. So light can, in truth, kill. If you're stuck in the Sahara without sun protection, even if you have water, you'll find that it can kill much faster.

Clearly, we can see that light can harm human tissues. Can it help them? Much of the initial research in this regard was done (in America, at least) by a man named John Ott. He was a banker by trade and a photographer by avocation until his banking got in the way of his photography. He quit banking to focus on his true love behind the camera, and was an early pioneer in time-lapse photography. He filmed many of Walt Disney's time-lapse flower-blooming scenes in the '50s and '60s.

At that early stage of the art, most time-lapse filming had to be done inside. Cameras weren't weatherproof and outside plants moved around too much from the effects of wind, weather, and sun position. So Ott experimented extensively with indoor lighting, and found that it varied to an astonishing degree in its effects on plants. Some killed the plants, some produced sickly specimens, and some was clearly healthy for them. Some light produced all male blossoms and some all female blossoms on monoecious (male and female blossom-producing) pumpkin plants.

Later, he found that some light would prevent fish in an aquarium from laying eggs, some would cause them to lay eggs, some would cause all female offspring, and some would cause majority (80 percent) male offspring. These findings were revolutionary at the time, and caused him to begin observing light's effects on humans. One especially useful finding he discovered (by accident) is particularly applicable to the subject of this report.

As he aged, he began to experience severe arthritis in his hip. It eventually necessitated his using a cane simply to walk, but his reliance on the cane became so extreme that he began to experience debilitating pain in his arm. Knowing that light was crucial for human health, he spent a great deal of time on the beach in Florida, but doing so was not helping him. His breakthrough came when he broke his sunglasses. He began to sit in the sun (not directly, but in the shade where he would get plenty of reflected sun) without his sunglasses.

In short order, his arthritis began to recede. He was soon able to throw away his cane, and shortly thereafter he was able to walk without a limp. His finding was that the ultraviolet rays of the sun, which are filtered out not only by sunglasses but by the glass in windows and even normal glasses, were essential for health. Without UV, a number of health problems can come up – certainly including arthritis.[36]

The upshot of all this is that if you suffer from arthritis (or any other inflammation-related disease), the second thing you should do, after adjusting your diet to eliminate simple carbs, is to spend lots of time in indirect sunlight without any glass between you and the light. If your vision is extremely bad and you require glasses to keep from stumbling, you should probably do this by

---

36   This information on John Ott and his work is summarized from two of his books, *Health and Light*, Devin-Adair, Publishers, Greenwich, Connecticut, 1973, and *Light, Radiation, & You*, Devin-Adair, 1982, 1990. These two books formed much of the basis for the study of the effects of light on health in the U.S.

sitting in the shade for as long as is comfortable. If you can see well enough without corrective lenses of any kind, I would suggest alternating sitting in this manner with activities in the sun such as walking, biking, or playing games such as tennis or volleyball. Fishing, swimming, hiking, or similar activities are also ideal. Let your imagination and your druthers be your guide. This is some of the cheapest and most pleasant medicine you'll ever employ – and perhaps some of the most beneficial. Just don't let a good thing become bad. Protect yourself from the damaging effects of the sun by limiting your exposure through clothing and shade. Sunblock tends to carry some of its own threats to health unless it's a natural brand, so it's normally not a good idea unless the alternative is burning.

The science for this process is fairly limited at this point in time. However, the risk is virtually zero, if you don't get a sunburn or too much heat. So your reward/risk ratio is potentially huge. I have no hesitation whatsoever in recommending such a procedure. Even if it does little to relieve your specific area of intense pain, it will leave your general health better for the experience. And the strong possibility exists that it will be of great help for your arthritis or inflammatory problem.

Light therapy goes far beyond cooling your heels in the shade, however. John Ott's work did much to prove that fact, and others have taken his work far beyond its auspicious beginnings.

Color Therapy

I include this section thanks largely to a wonderful man of medical science, William Campbell Douglass, M.D., whom I worked with for much of the 1990s. I was the first editor of his medical newsletter when it launched in 1991, and found him to be a man concerned with true science and true healing.

He wrote a book titled *Into the Light*,[37] which I worked on with him. Much of the book is dedicated to the ultraviolet irradiation of blood, which we will discuss in a later section of this chapter. However, he also discussed the concept of color therapy (also called chromo-therapy), or Spectro-Chrome therapy, as it was called by its developer, Dinshah Ghadiali.[38] In practice, color therapy has evidenced strong potential to affect human health for the better. In theory, it sounds – well, it just sounds strange to many people. To address this dichotomy, and perhaps to put this therapy and one or two others I'll discuss later in an understandable (for most Americans) context, permit me to digress a moment.

As Mr. Ghadiali's name implies, he was Indian in ancestry – though he did much of his work on light therapy in America. While he left India behind, he brought with him much of the Hindu framework that organized his life in India. His work with light therefore combined an empirical summary of what exposing patients to different wavelengths of light accomplished with

37   Second Opinion Publishing, Inc., Dunwoody, GA, 1993.
38   You can read more about Ghadiali's work at DinshahHealth.org.

a theory of causation rooted in his Hindu worldview. Wikipedia's entry on chromotherapy shows much of what this looks or sounds like when a typical practitioner explains it. The treatment is tightly interwoven with Hindu thinking and concepts. This may give some readers pause, though I'm sure others will be comfortable with it.

This joining of color therapy with Hindu precepts appears to present Americans with a choice – a choice that is in fact a false dilemma. The choice appears to be that they can either accept color therapy and concurrently endorse, or at least tacitly accept, Hindu positions on the nature of reality, or throw the baby out with the bath water. This is an extremely unfortunate development.

Many Americans have deeply held religious convictions of their own that preclude any such endorsement or acceptance of Hindu concepts. Other, more secular, Americans question why they should accept health advice from a belief system that has produced a life expectancy among its adherents more than 10 years shorter than that of Americans.

None of this is to pass judgment on Hinduism or its prescriptions for living. Rather, it is to point out the error inherent in joining a healing therapy to a religion. This error is a serious one, and has resulted in color therapy being largely rejected in America. It is time for this therapy to stand on its own merits. It is not a Hindu therapy.[39] It is a therapy, period. It must stand or fall on that basis alone, even as Hinduism must stand or fall as a religion on its own merits alone. They are unconnected in any necessary or substantive way.

Many current alternative therapies are being explained in religious terms. Doing so effectively demands that they be judged on different criteria than conventional treatments. This seems to many people to be an admission that they can't compete on the same playing field with conventional treatments. To the extent that they can't compete on the field of corrupt, industrialized, crony capitalist mercantilism, that's a good thing. To the extent they can't compete on an objective scientific basis in which simple efficacy is the gold standard, it's a very bad thing. What I'm asking is that you evaluate color therapy and all other therapies in this report on a strict basis of efficacy: Do they work?

Despite their subservience to and abuse by crony capitalism[40] in America for years, Western concepts of energy production and use throughout the body are far more explanatory, useful, and predictive than Eastern concepts. Energy doesn't flow throughout the body (as in the Chinese concept of qi) or have energy centers within the body (chakras) or create an aura around a person. Rather, energy is produced within the cells in a way that is relatively well

---

39 Mr. Ghadiali's Hinduism doubtless caused him to be open to color therapy, even as Americans' Western mindset may have closed them off to such thinking. Nevertheless, the therapy itself is in no way dependent on Hindu positions of reality, and is not at odds with known physical and biological facts – though it has yet to be fully explained using those facts.
40 Crony capitalism isn't capitalist at all. It's the eliminating of competition by large corporations that pay off government legislators and regulators to get favorable treatment.

understood.[41] However, both blood and lymph circulate (flow) through the body, and they carry crucial nutrients and infection-fighting elements to the cells. By improving what they think is the flow of energy, many practitioners improve the flow of the fuel used for energy production and white blood cells used for fighting infection. That's an extremely beneficial outcome. Also, by their insistence on restoring optimum physiological normalcy, these practitioners pave the way for the body to operate more efficiently and with less pain. Aiming for the wrong target still hits a bull's-eye in this case. "Trying to improve the flow of energy" is a misconception of the process at work, but it still improves health.

So, with that introduction, we come to color therapy. As Western scientist and doctor W.C. Douglass has clinically proved, color therapy can be a very, very cheap way to attain highly substantive *results*. For that reason, it's something you should be aware of and look into.

The treatment is simple; you put the appropriate color of filter over the face of the light source, turn on the light, and shine the colored light on the skin over the diseased or painful part of the body. Ken Adachi writes in his "Educate Yourself" article on color therapy that:

> "Roscolene plastic color gels (filters) seem to work just as well [as Ghadiali's glass filters], and they are easier to obtain and carry around. [Darius Dinshah's book] *Let There Be Light* explains how to match the symptoms the patient is experiencing with the appropriate color filter(s) for a "tonation," as Dinshah had coined the treatment. Tonations are usually one hour long and the colored light is directed at the area of the body requiring treatment (all detailed in the book)."[42]

As Dr. Douglass says,

oscillations

> "The idea of shining a specific color on a diseased part of the body for treatment will sound preposterous to most, but think about it: ultraviolet and infrared, both invisible parts of the electromagnetic spectrum, are readily recognized as useful in medicine, so why should anyone be surprised that the rest of the spectrum, i.e., visible light, is also useful? Applications of light — the color red, for instance, which has a frequency of 436,803,079,680,000 oscillations per second – is just as much a form of energy as the note high C, which has an oscillation frequency of 4,096 oscillations per second. X-rays, gamma-rays, delta-rays, and magnetism are all forms of oscillatory energy. As far as we know, magnetism has the highest oscillatory rate, which is 18,446,744,073,709,551,616 oscillations per second...."

I am dragging you through all of these numbers to help you understand colors are not what

---

41 Nerves seem to conduct their messages to the spinal cord and brain via electrical impulses, but they are more analogous to telephone lines than power lines. They carry messages via small amounts of electrical current, not huge quantities of current to power the homes and offices of end users.

42 Adachi K. Dinshah P. Ghadiali & Spectro-Chrome Therapy. Educate Yourself. 2001. http://educate-yourself.org/products/dinshahandspectrochrome.shtml. Accessed August 16, 2013.

you *see*, but what they *are*: vibratory energy.[43]

Mr. Ghadiali and some of his students cured cases deemed hopeless by conventional medicine. These cases included severe burns, a case of colitis that nearly killed its victim, and advanced pulmonary tuberculosis that was on the verge of killing a young boy. Clearly, in many cases, color therapy works, and works well. How? I'm not at all certain, unless you accept that the electromagnetic energy from colored light works on the energy aura surrounding human beings.[44] I'm not there yet. If you are, so be it. Just try the therapy. It's too cheap and safe an option not to give it a try.

Color therapy was reported to be making rapid inroads into conventional medical practice in the US until the American Medical Association (AMA) became alarmed. As a non-patentable, inexpensive procedure, color therapy was apparently quite a threat to cartel income, so the AMA brought suit against Mr. Ghadiali in court. *Ghadiali won*, but the proceedings, with accompanying media prattle, tainted the procedure in the public mind – which was doubtless the intent, win or lose in court. One of Ghadiali's chief supporting witnesses was a medical doctor named Kate Baldwin, who had used color therapy extensively and to amazing effect.

Dr. Baldwin submitted a paper to the clinical meeting of the Section on Eye, Ear, Nose, and Throat Diseases of the Medical Society of the State of Pennsylvania on October 12, 1926.[45] (As you see, this occurred a long time ago, but the qualities of light and those of disease or injury have not changed in nearly 90 years – or in thousands of years, for that matter.)

"For about six years, I have given close attention to the action of colors in restoring the body functions, and I am perfectly honest in saying that, after nearly 37 years of active hospital and private practice in medicine and surgery, I can produce quicker and more accurate results with colors than with any or all other methods combined – and with less strain on the patient. In many cases, the functions have been restored after the classical remedies have failed. Of course, surgery is necessary in some cases, but results will be quicker and better if color is used before and after operation. Sprains, bruises, and traumata of all sorts respond to color as to no other treatment. Septic conditions yield, regardless of the specific organism. Cardiac lesions, asthma, hay fever, pneumonia, inflammatory conditions of the eyes, corneal ulcers, glaucoma, and cataracts are relieved by the treatment.

"The treatment of carbuncles [large, oozing boils] with color is easy compared to the classical methods. One woman with a carbuncle involving the back of the neck from mastoid to mastoid, and from occipital ridge to the first dorsal vertebra, came under color

---

43 *Into the Light*, 224-225.
44 A more likely explanation has to do with resonance frequencies that both enhance the health of the body's cells and degrade the operation of or kill infectious organisms. This is explained in more detail in the section on FSM.
45 *Atlanta Medical Journal*, April 1927, as quoted in *Into the Light*, 292-293.

therapy after ten days of the very best of attention. From the first day of color application, no opiates, not even sedatives, were required. This patient was saved much suffering, and she has little scar.

"The use of color in the treatment of burns is well worth investigation by every member of the professions. In such cases, the burning sensation caused by the destructive forces may be counteracted in from 20 to 30 minutes, and it does not return. True burns are caused by the destructive action of the red side of the spectrum, hydrogen predominating. Apply oxygen by the use of the blue side of the spectrum, and much will be done to relieve the nervous strain, the healing processes are rapid, and the resulting tissues soft and flexible."

Within the scope of my two decades of experience and research, color therapy has a zero medical risk factor. That's not a rounded number. It's zero. Period. Your risk is limited to the money you put out for the filter system, your time, the possibility that the therapy will not work for you,[46] and possibly your dignity if you go talking about this to skeptics (so don't do that).

Light therapy is therefore one of the most efficacious, inexpensive, and simple therapies you can avail yourself of. To ignore it could be a serious mistake, regardless of its strangeness in a Western medical context or its past grounding in Eastern religion. *It is a physical phenomenon with demonstrated biological effects.* Look at it and use it that way. By experimenting with it, you can easily become an expert in its administration and help everyone in your family and even your friends and acquaintances.

One other point to consider is that Dr. Baldwin, Dr. Douglass, and others who make extensive use of light therapy often quote cases in which rapid response to the therapy occurred. That is not always the case, even for them. Such cases prove the usefulness of the therapy, and they happen often, but they're not always typical. Light therapy is a gentle therapy, though clearly powerful. It often takes some time to work. So prepare your mind and your schedule to allow several sessions of light therapy. If they're not necessary, you'll have your schedule back – and most people can always put *more* time to good use.

If you go to shokos.com/LightIndex.htm, you'll find a link and/or a phone number to order their most popular light kit for $82 (at this writing) plus shipping. It contains a book on color therapy by Mr. Ghadiali's son (who adopted Ghadiali's given name as his surname), Darius Dinshah, a light fixture to which a filter holder can be attached, and 26 colored filters. With this kit and a filter holder, available for $4, you can administer a very wide range of therapeutic light colors, which treat an even wider array of conditions. If you just want to put the filters over a flashlight or a desk lamp you have at home, you can get a set of 26 6½" square filters for $41 plus shipping.

---

46   Strictly speaking, this can be a medical risk factor in that trying a procedure that doesn't work can delay trying another that might work. But light therapy is usually the last thing tried because most people just don't think it will work. For serious injuries or wounds, that's definitely how you should proceed – at least until you've established your own skill with the therapy and know its – and your – limits.

Infrared Sauna

Infrared (IR) saunas are becoming quite popular now, and many companies offer them for sale. They are not cheap, typically costing several thousand dollars, so they are not for everyone.

The historical sauna employed bricks or stones heated to 180-200°F, on which water was poured, creating steam. The small wooden room within which this occurred would thereby be heated, as well, and the persons within would sweat out toxins in their bodies. In Scandinavia, where the concept originated, this would often suffice for a bath in the winter months, and would soothe tired muscles and joints while doing a fairly substantial detox. After working all day in temperatures ranging from minus 20 to minus 50, this was doubtlessly an extremely welcome and invigorating process.

The IR sauna does essentially the same thing, but is simpler and requires less heating of the air within the sauna. No steam is produced, rather IR light is emitted, which heats the skin and underlying tissue to a depth of up to half a centimeter. IR light *is* heat, and all things that emit heat are emitting IR light. It is because of this fact that thermal imaging equipment can allow one to see heat-emitting entities, such as people, animals, or stoves or ovens, through walls, at night, or through fog. Such equipment is simply a receptor for IR light, and converts an IR signature into a visible light picture for human viewing.

Most saunas claim to use what is called "far infrared" light, which is invisible to the eye, and has a 5.5 to 15 micron (micrometer, or μm) wavelength. (One μm is one-millionth of a meter, while one nanometer, or nm, is one-billionth of a meter.) Consider that the IR spectrum includes near (700-800 nm), short-wavelength (1.4-3 μm), mid (3-8 μm), and long IR (8-15 μm) wavelengths of light.[47] However, Walter Crinnion, ND, who uses IR sauna in his practice, claims that all IR saunas emit wavelengths from all IR bands while in operation.

IR saunas are approved by the FDA for pain, and have been used for many conditions. That said, they have not been used long enough to exhaustively test their utility. Significant disagreement exists on what wavelength of IR light is best for therapy, and how best to use them. The matter is primarily being disputed in marketing ads for one company versus another – which is not necessarily the best forum for obtaining objective information.

Studies are being done, however. One study found IR saunas useful in treating rheumatoid arthritis and ankylosing spondylitis (the stiffening or fusing of bones caused by inflammation, typically in the vertebrae).[48] Only eight sauna treatments were administered over four weeks, but the patients experienced significant relief from their inflammation-related pain.

Other conditions that have been treated with varying degrees of success include acne;

---

47 Infrared light. RP Photonics Encyclopedia. http://www.rp-photonics.com/infrared_light.html. Accessed August 16, 2013.
48 Oosterveld FGJ, Rasker JJ, Floors M, et al, Infrared sauna in patients with rheumatoid arthritis and ankylosing spondylitis. *Clin Rheumatol*. 2009;(28):29–34.

cancer (for detoxification and improved uptake of cancer-cell-killing substances); soft-tissue injury; menstrual pain; eczema; upper respiratory infections; wound healing; Bell's palsy; neurodermatitis; GI problems; cardiovascular diseases; hypertension; and ear, nose, and throat disorders such as sore throat, chronic middle ear inflammation, and infection.[49]

Doctors who use IR saunas in treatment protocols often use an extensive list of therapies, including exercise, diet, dietary supplements, and sometimes other detoxification methods. An article by Dr. Crinnion can be downloaded within the report of "Proceedings from the 13th International Symposium of the Institute for Functional Medicine."[50] He lists his own protocol there, as well as a less extensive one used by L. Ron Hubbard of Scientology fame (if you have an unpleasant reaction to that reference, remember what I said earlier about therapies standing on their own merits). Both resulted in very significant detoxification effects, and Dr. Crinnion's protocol resulted in (using his very subjective grading scale) from "slight" to "great" improvement in all patients treated for musculoskeletal issues.

The upshot of this therapy appears to be that it offers temporary relief from joint and muscle pain if you use it by itself. If you use it with other things such as diet and exercise, it seems to expedite and magnify the results. In short, I would recommend buying one primarily if you enjoy sauna for its own sake – not because it doesn't work therapeutically, but because it provides effects that can be obtained less expensively with other modalities. A sauna provides a very pleasant experience (I speak from experience of the traditional Finnish sauna), so if you enjoy it enough to purchase it for that reason, you will likely enjoy some (and possibly a highly) therapeutic benefit in regard to skin, muscle, joint, nerve, and detox issues.

Also, as quantified in the earlier cited study published in *Clinical Rheumatology*, a sauna increases the heart rate commensurate with the temperature of the sauna. A sauna has an effect very similar to exercise. So if for any reason you can't exercise, you can get basically the same effect you'd get in exercising with oxygen by breathing oxygen in a sauna (see Chapter 12). This procedure is being experimented with, and initial results are promising. There appears to be no downside to it, as long as there is no possibility of open flame or spark in the sauna. Oxygen, of course, mixes with flame explosively.

Polarized Light Therapy

This therapy will be a little more difficult to cover than others due to the structure of its industry. For all intents and purposes, only one company provides devices that emit polarized light for medical treatments. The company is Zepter (its products are known by the name of a subordinate company, Bioptron). The polarized light device was invented by a physician in Budapest, Hungary, and the rights to it purchased by Bioptron in 1986.

---

49   Rader A. Hot stuff.
50   Components of practical clinical detox programs – sauna as a therapeutic tool. 2006:S154-S156. Downloadable at alternative-therapies.com/at/web_pdfs/ifm_proceedings_low.pdf#page=76.

Polarized light is light that has been unified in its directional wave characteristics. Normal light has light that oscillates in every direction. To visualize what this means, imagine a car traveling a non-curving road over hill and valley. It goes up and down as it travels, but does not go right or left. Now imagine a car on the salt flats in Utah, but on a road that regularly curves right and left. It doesn't go up and down, but it goes right and left. Light is like this, except that it oscillates in every imaginable plane, not just vertical or horizontal. When you polarize light, you block all light that oscillates in a plane other than the one you choose. So, for instance, all the light you allow to pass a polarizing lens might oscillate up and down. Nothing else gets through.

Polarized sunglasses do this, allowing light with only one wave orientation to get through. Polarized light is also used in photography (the inventor of polarized lenses called them Polaroids), liquid crystal displays (LCDs), microscopy, and many other purposes used in medicine and science.

Since Bioptron is the only company in this field, we have little information about its products or technology from anywhere but the company itself. That's not necessarily an indication that the information is bad, but it is a factor to consider.

That said, I became interested in polarized light therapy because of an article I read on it in the 1990s. I procured one of Bioptron's devices, and my family and I have used it on several occasions. It has been very helpful in the treatment of many soft tissue injuries, and its use on my back has been significant, as well. I have not used it extensively enough to know if it aids in long-term healing, but it provides relief when pain flares up.

The injuries for which this device seems to be most well-adapted are soft tissue injuries or problems. The penetration of the light is sufficient and beneficial for things such as burns, skin conditions, venous leg ulcers, surgical incisions, and other painful skin conditions, along with muscle injuries and, to a lesser extent, joint injuries.

According to the company, the device essentially does for the skin and deeper tissues what some of the oxygen and prolotherapy treatments do for joints and muscles – it stimulates circulation and brings increased blood flow and oxygenation to the tissues. This increases cellular energy, increases protein synthesis (collagen and elastin production), and reduces swelling and inflammation.

The device is used in treating both osteo- and rheumatoid arthritis; neck, shoulder, and lower back pain; carpal tunnel syndrome; musculoskeletal injuries; sprains, strains, contusions, and tendonitis; and ligament and muscle tears.

I'll add something of a postscript to this section by noting that my wife has been treating a peculiar numbness and muscle dysfunction in her right wrist and hand with our Bioptron device. In her initial irradiations, of about 10 minutes each, nothing seemed to be happening. However, in order to give a better tryout to the device for this report, she stuck with it. After several days of treatment, this longstanding problem (of over a year at this writing) has been resolving for her. She has experienced more relief than she has had in months. It has not completely resolved at this writing, but indications are good. It's important to say that, as with many light therapies, the treatment is gentle and gradual. Results might not be apparent immediately. The company's Web site is bioptron.com. You can find a distributor by calling 201-453-0637 or emailing info@zepter-usa.com.

Laser Therapy

Lasers are now a well-known form of light that finds application in a number of ways. Laser pointers are common; CDs and DVDs are played by lasers; wood, metal, and glass can be laser etched or carved by laser; and the list goes on. Some forms of delicate, precise surgery are also accomplished by laser, such as eye surgery.

The physics of laser light are not easy to explain. Suffice it to say that laser light is monochromatic (one color), coherent (the peaks and valleys of each wave are lined up like a phalanx of well-trained soldiers), and directional (all photon emissions in the beam are travelling in close parallel – precisely in the same direction – again, like a phalanx of well-trained soldiers). These characteristics cause lasers to be very tightly focused at any distance from the emitting source, and very intense. Accordingly, whatever the characteristics of the wavelength of light being used, they are multiplied in a laser.

The following table[51] provides a simple comparison of light wavelengths characteristic of lasers emitted from various source materials.

Laser Type	Wavelength (nm)
Argon fluoride (UV)	193
Krypton fluoride (UV)	248
Xenon chloride (UV)	308
Nitrogen (UV)	337
Argon (blue)	488
Argon (green)	514
Helium neon (green)	543
Helium neon (red)	633
Rhodamine 6G dye (tunable)	570-650
Ruby ($CrAlO_3$) (red)	694
Nd:Yag (NIR)	1064
Carbon dioxide (FIR)	10600

---

51   Weschler M. How lasers work. Howstuffworks. http://science.howstuffworks.com/laser4.htm. Accessed September 7, 2013.

Notice that the wavelength of a laser emanating from carbon dioxide is in the far-infrared region of the invisible light spectrum (10,600 nm = 10.6 μm), as explained in the section on IR saunas. Recall that infrared light is heat, and imagine what happens when you tightly concentrate and cause to cohere the light from an intense IR light source. Such a laser is extremely potent, and can cut through steel. It is a very dangerous laser – albeit highly useful when properly contained.

This is further evidence of light's effects on various substances. If anyone tells you that light doesn't have any effect, ask them how it can cut through steel. But that's an extreme. The beautiful thing about light is that it comes in a spectrum. You can see some of that spectrum anytime you look at a rainbow, but the full spectrum of electromagnetic radiation, which is the category that includes visible light, is much, much broader (see figure below[52]). Therefore, if one wavelength of light is too strong or weak, another might be just right.

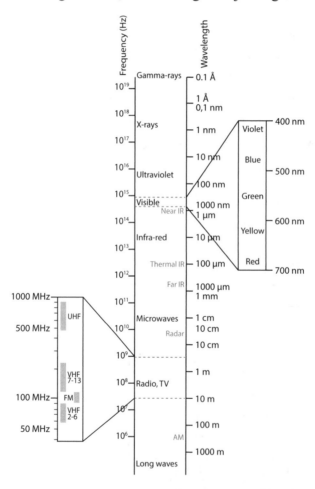

When it comes to therapeutic lasers, just right turns out to be in the range of 600 to 1000 nm. This is the red to near infrared range. Some lasers have been produced for therapeutic uses outside of this range, but this is where most of the lasers being used medically operate at this writing.

---

52   Image from Wikipedia Commons: https://commons.wikimedia.org/wiki/Main_Page

Low Level Laser Therapy

One form of laser therapy is low-level laser treatment (LLLT). This is a favorite therapy of Dr. Robert Rowen, a practicing doctor and well-known writer. He discovered it at a medical symposium, and used it on his own very painful skiing injury, to quick and thorough effect. That injury, to his shoulder, had failed to heal for weeks, and quickly resolved with the use of the laser.[53]

The laser is a small, handheld device. Its light penetrates only about two inches, which nevertheless stimulates substantial healing in deep tissues. It has a wavelength of 635 nm – ideal, according to clinical studies, for both healing and for killing bacteria in wounds and injuries. The power needed is miniscule – only 5 milliwatts or less.

The laser is intended to penetrate the body to a deeper level than most visible light. It imparts its energy to the cells in the body, which stimulates thousands of chemical reactions there. This results in something called biological amplification, which causes an increase in the rate of healing.

In an Indian study rats were cut on either side of their backbone.[54] Both sides were immediately cleaned and sutured, and one side was treated with laser. The other side was not exposed to laser. Mean healing time was five days on the treated side, compared to seven days on the untreated side. Perhaps more important, however, the wounds on the treated side were found to be significantly stronger and more resistant to re-injury. The laser used in this study was a helium-neon (He-Ne) laser of 5 mw and 633 nm wavelength, very close to the ideal of 635 nm.

Further, the researchers found that, "Although the effect of He-Ne laser on wound healing is predominantly local, its biostimulatory effect can be seen in the contralateral nonirradiated side as well."[55] In other words, both wounds on each rat appeared to benefit from the laser treatment, though only one was exposed. The researchers do not elaborate, but perhaps the effects of the laser could be better seen in two subjects with one wound each (one treated with laser, the other not) rather than one subject with two wounds.

In his practice, Dr. Rowen noted several instances in which wounds were rapidly healed using LLLT. One woman dropped a 45-pound weight on her foot at the gym, resulting in serious bruising and swelling. After five laser treatments overnight, the blackness, swelling, and pain had greatly receded and she could walk again. She was running and working out in tennis shoes within two days of the injury. Within three days, after continued treatments, the effects of the injury were almost gone.

A middle-aged couple used the laser to heal herpes lesions within three days (normal

---

53   *Second Opinion*, January 2007.
54   Bisht D, Mehrotra R, Singh PA, et al. Effect of helium-neon laser on wound healing. *Indian J Exp Biol.* 1999;37(2):187-189.
55   Ibid., 188.

healing took 10 to 12 days). A 62-year-old ex-pro baseball player with severe sciatica was treated one time in a doctor's office and walked out with no pain. He bought a laser to maintain the effects of the treatment.

A woman suffered from horrible headaches, caused by an infected tooth, for 16 years. Her dentist couldn't figure out what to do to stop it. She tried a laser on the tooth, and "it penetrated right through her maxillary bone to the root of the problem. Her pain was gone in seconds."[56] This result was possible because a laser in the wavelength of 630 nm has strong antibacterial properties. The infecting bacteria in her tooth were literally killed off in a very short period of time, which in turn killed her pain.

Initial lasers of this type were quite large. They worked well, but the FDA shut down the manufacture of them before many could be sold. The new laser used in all these cases is quite a bit smaller. It looks like, and is the size of, a high-tech, high-quality remote for your TV, but it emits two or four beams of "light amplification by stimulated emission of radiation" (LASER). Its inventor, Dr. Gerry Graham, obtained FDA approval for his device.

You can find information at lazrpulsr.com or you can call 888-696-6532. At this writing, the two-laser basic consumer model costs $2,995. The two-laser consumer model with greater programming for more conditions costs $4,995. The four-laser professional model costs $7,495, and a more capable professional model is in the works. The company is working on constructing a Web page featuring contact information for professionals who will treat you at their offices using this device (accessible via the "Find a Clinic Near You" tab at the lazrpulsr.com home page), but the page is not available at this writing. When complete, this page will offer a significant advantage. You'll be able to try out the therapy at a professional's office for far less than the cost of a device. If it works for you, you can then decide whether to spring for a device of your own.

High Power Laser Therapy

LLLT lasers are not the only option for medical laser therapy. Many doctors and chiropractors have incorporated lasers into their practices. They are typically of a type that provides what is called High Power Laser Therapy (HPLT). They are known as Class IV lasers (LLLT lasers are Class III lasers). My chiropractor offers laser treatments with a brand new, state-of-the-art Class IV laser for $20 per treatment. It had significant efficacy for me when the doctor did the treatment himself, but when he turned it over to his assistant the benefit was negligible. This, I suspect, was an issue of laser proximity to the problem area.

My doctor irradiated my spine from the front (which he asserts, and my experience supports, treats lower back problems better). He placed the laser at the belt-line, left of center (from my perspective), and pressed *hard*. The reason he did that was that the laser is able to

56   Rowen. January 2007.

penetrate only a few inches of soft tissue. This is quite a bit further than most light can penetrate, but it's still a limitation when trying to reach the spine from the front. My doctor's assistant, whether from lack of strength, fear of hurting me, inexperience, or failure to understand the importance of placing the laser tip close to the spine, did not press hard enough. The benefit to me of her treatments was negligible as a result.

This anecdote illustrates both the efficacy of laser treatments and the sometimes-tricky nature of getting the light where it needs to be. The body's complexity (or excess weight) can thwart the most well-intentioned of proven therapies, and make them seem worthless. Hence the importance of educating yourself on human physiology and biology, and talking with others who have expertise in the field. Perhaps just as important – often more important – it's critical to try many ways of doing a thing before concluding it's not working. If at first you don't succeed….

Class IV lasers use light with wavelengths in the range of 810 to 890 nm. This is a longer wavelength than the LLLT lasers, in the near infrared range. However, the wavelengths are still in a fairly cool range of operation (relatively little heat emission), so heat damage is not a problem with a knowledgeable practitioner. (My doctor simply told me to let him know when it felt hot. Eventually it did, but not excessively. He then stopped when I indicated that I was beginning to feel heat.) Many professional athletes undergo laser therapy of this type, which is currently better known and more common than LLLT. It provides them pain reduction, tissue and nerve repair, and functional recovery faster and to a greater extent than traditional treatments.

Companies with these devices market them for conditions as varied as peripheral neuropathy; head, neck, and back pain (stenosis, disc herniations, and sciatica); arthritis; carpal tunnel syndrome; foot and heel pain; ligament and tendon injuries; muscle bruising; and non-healing wounds. Their lasers are prohibitively expensive for personal purchase – my doctor's device cost well north of $40,000. However, as is the case with my doctor, getting a treatment in the office might be well within budget for most of us. Such costs make trying the treatment out very easy to do. (The only challenge is getting an appointment. At that cost, his laser is busy all day every day, and is scheduled weeks in advance.)

Ultraviolet Blood Irradiation (UBI) Therapy

Ultraviolet light might seem to be a strange thing to mention in the context of blood therapy. After all, UV light kills microorganisms on exposure, and blood cells are very similar in many respects to microorganisms (they're small and living). But it turns out that short-term exposure to the range of light called ultraviolet C (UV C), which is the germicidal range, is not harmful to blood. It's very harmful, however, for viruses and bacteria.

The therapy consists of withdrawing small amounts of blood from the body (as little as a syringe-full, though significantly more is typically used). This blood sample is exposed to UV C light, then reintroduced to the body. In the earliest experiments, the thinking was that, since UV light kills viruses and bacteria, running the entire blood supply out of the body, through a brief exposure to a UV light source, and back into the body (a little at a time, of course) would kill whatever ailed a person. Had it been done on people, it would instead have killed the person. It did kill the lab animals on which it was tested.

The researchers regrouped and retested, exposing only a little of the blood to UV light. The results were astounding, and of a completely different nature than expected. Rather than killing the infecting organisms directly, the light instead stimulated the body's immune system. And the amount of stimulation was immense. After exposure and reinjection of the blood, the immune system was able to throw off incredibly serious infections and even such things as toxins from snakes and other venomous animals.

Polio was healed with the therapy, as were thrombophlebitis (infection of the veins), septicemia (blood poisoning), botulism, gas gangrene, Staphylococcus, and even bronchial pneumonia. What this means for you as you struggle with pain is that any pain related to bacterial or viral infection, or to some sort of toxin, can likely be alleviated or greatly reduced with the use of UBI.

People with septic toxemia, which is a bacterial infection in the blood, often experience related headache, muscle ache, and other types of pain. This condition responds so well to UBI that patients are often pain-free before the treatment is complete.[57]

Cases of infectious arthritis, cerebral thrombosis, various skin conditions, viral pneumonia, and mumps have been healed by UBI.[58] It has broad utility for many conditions that have an infectious cause. In fact, as pharmaceutical companies begin to lose interest in producing new strains of antibiotics due to "inadequate profitability" and old strains lose their effectiveness due to antibiotic-resistance, UBI might finally start getting some of the respect it deserves.

If you suffer from pain that has an infectious disease or toxic source,[59] try UBI. You can find a practitioner at acamnet.org. Scroll down about halfway on the page to the "Locate an ACAM Physician" line. Put in your zip code and conduct a search. You can widen your search to your state or neighboring state by going to "More Search Options." UBI practitioners will be listed as having a specialty in "Photoluminescence," another name for UBI.

---

57   Douglass W. *Into the Light.* Second Opinion Publishing, Inc., Dunwoody, GA, 1993. P. 96.
58   *Into the Light.* Pp. 19, 21, 29, 69-70, 100-102.
59   This applies to toxins from living sources such as bacterial infections, snakes, or spiders, not environmental toxins such as heavy metals or chemicals.

Chapter 11

Magnetic Therapy

Basic Magnets

Magnets are like bumble bees, whose wings are too small for flight. Magnets can't work. There is no mechanism of action yet proposed that will satisfy a serious scientist that they can reduce pain. Yet hundreds of thousands of people use them and say they work – evidence, say scientists, of the gullibility of man. "Placebo effect. Pure quackery. Nothing more."

This, of course, from people who believe that chemotherapy is good, cholesterol is bad, hospitals are safe, and government-licensed doctors are all driven by the noblest of motives.

Back to magnets. I can't tell you why they work. I can't even tell you categorically *that* they work. I can only tell you that lots of folks think they work, many studies from Eastern Europe show they work,[60] a very good study from America shows they work, and lots of serious doctors have used them for patients, and report that they work.

I've used them, and I've experienced relief. Significant relief. Not healing, but relief. Of course, this was for my back, and using permanent magnets on an injury like that is not really expected to be curative. But I felt better, and, given the pain I live with, I'll take it.

With all of that said, I'm not convinced that magnets' only positive contribution is a placebo effect. No one knows how they work. Every proffered explanation can be shot down in flames by a knowledgeable scientist. Trying to convince them of its validity is like leading with your chin in a fist fight. Further, it's true that many people have used claims about magnetism to commit outright fraud (such as claiming that paper, leather, and fabrics have been magnetized). But I still acknowledge physical phenomena beyond human understanding (not necessarily mystical, just as-yet unknown). And I suspect such a thing in the use of true magnets for therapeutic purposes.

Fifteen years ago, a key and well-conducted study at Baylor University found that magnets had a highly pronounced effect on pain in people who had had polio. The study was double-blinded, very well set-up and monitored, and *strongly* indicative of very substantive efficacy with magnets. The differences in pain reduction between those who used magnets and those who didn't were quite large. Few studies have been done since then, and some that have (such

---

60 Summaries of 120 studies done with static magnetic fields in Eastern Europe show frequent significant clinical effects. Studies summarized were divided between animal and human studies, controlled and uncontrolled. Human studies included research on burns, carpal tunnel syndrome, endometriosis, fractures, and polyneuritis. Jerabek J, Pawluk W. *Magnetic Therapy in Eastern Europe: A Review of 30 Years of Research*. 2009. 149-164.

as sleeping on a magnetic mattress, which also indicated benefit with magnets) were impossible to monitor to make sure patients weren't determining whether they had magnets or a placebo (a simple paper clip or a bobby pin can be a spoiler in such studies). Still, there's now some very interesting science on this topic.

I recommend that you give magnets a try. Don't get the ridiculously expensive ones – one thing the establishment know-it-alls have right is that the field is ripe for charlatans and exaggerators. When a thing is not understood, all kind of claims can be made for it, and marketers go wild with magnets.

Try some basic magnets that you can apply to your pain site in a form-fitted way, and make sure you have the right poles against your body. It shouldn't matter which way they're facing, as the skeptics are fond of reminding us, but it does. People who work with magnets know that one side works better than the other. If you're going to take the plunge and try magnets, take the plunge and orient them correctly. Any good set of medical magnets will have instructions on which side to place against your body, and many products have the magnets set in a band or dressing that positions them correctly.

If you want to use magnets from the store, get some that are flat and adhesive tape them or Ace bandage them to your skin. Apply the negative pole against your skin. You can determine the pole with a magnetometer if you just happen to have one lying around. If not, the north indicator of a compass needle points to the negative pole of a magnet and away from the positive pole.[61] Use a cheap compass for this determination, as this process can damage a compass.

Pulsed Electro-Magnetic Field

If you've studied magnets very much, you know that they can be created either by permanently orienting the domains within the magnetic material, or they can be temporarily created by running an electrical current through a wire wrapped around the material. In a permanent magnet or an electromagnet powered by direct current (DC), the magnetic field is static. In an electromagnet powered by alternating current (AC), the resulting magnetic field is referred to as time varying. The current waxes and wanes many times every second, depending on the frequency of the current being passed through it.

This kind of electromagnetic current turns out to have extensive application to chronic diseases and injuries, as well as the pain that arises from them. This application has been studied extensively, but not in America. The derision heaped upon magnetic field therapy in the US has precluded very much research on the subject until relatively recently. But a great deal of research has been done in Eastern Europe.

---

61   Magnetic field therapy. Alternative Medicine Therapies. http://library.thinkquest.org/24206/magnetic-field-ther-apy.html. Accessed August 16, 2013.

In the USSR, and in Eastern Europe after the USSR's fall, using the extremely expensive procedures and drugs used in the US usually wasn't possible. The government couldn't afford to fund such a system, so it turned to procedures that offered a great deal of bang for the buck – or ruble, as it were. Ultraviolet blood irradiation, pioneered in the US, was one such therapy that attained a significant degree of acceptability in the USSR. But another treatment the Eastern Bloc countries researched and used extensively was pulsed electro-magnetic field (PEMF) therapy.

A couple of English-speaking medical doctors who also know Eastern-bloc languages compiled the results of 343 studies done on PEMF in Russia and Eastern Europe over the past 30 years.[62] These studies would be difficult to confirm based on the language barrier, the diversity of origins of the studies (done in many countries), and the fact that either they were unpublished or publication information was not included. With such factors involved, the possibility of inaccuracy or even invention cannot be ruled out. However, the summaries are quite detailed and feature information that would be difficult to fabricate. They cannot be given the same weight as expert-reviewed (I use the term "expert" rather than "peer" because peers are not always the best critics) study write-ups, but they are useful as adjuncts to other information known about PEMF. They strongly suggest that substantive, extensive, and varied research has been done in Eastern Europe over the course of several decades – which is the claim made for this therapy.

Included in the research were a number of disease states. Specifically related to pain, the researchers studied soft tissue inflammation, vertebral pain syndromes, ankylosing spondylitis, osteoarthritis, rheumatoid arthritis, and low back pain. The authors observed that, "...static magnetic fields should be used in patients with severe acute conditions, if magnetic therapy is suitable at all. In chronic diseases time-varying fields are more suitable."[63] It is therefore perhaps not surprising that static-field magnets have had only a temporary relief effect with my chronic back problem.

Use of PEMF typically involved 20-30 minute sessions for 10 exposures, usually one treatment per day. All categories except arthritis experienced strong improvements in pain relief and healing times. Osteoarthritis was treated with a combination of hydrotherapy and PEMF, so the particular contribution of PEMF was not determined. That said, the results were strongly positive. With regard to rheumatoid arthritis, mild to moderate cases did well. Severe cases involved worsening of the disease before any improvement occurred.

Dr. Rowen uses PEMF on himself and his patients, but also had his dad buy a top-of-the-line machine. His dad groused about having to spend so much money, and wanted to sell it after treating (and resolving) the initial problem for which he bought it. But then he realized what all it was doing for him. Dr. Rowen notes that, "He is using it for his prostate, back pain, macular degeneration, and overall rejuvenation. My dad, at 94, is improving by leaps and bounds in strength, gait, cognitive function, and pain levels. My eye-surgeon sister, who saw him recently,

62 *Magnetic Therapy in Eastern Europe*; 149-164.
63 *Magnetic Therapy in Eastern Europe*; 165.

says he's even seen an improvement in his urinary function. This is largely unheard of for a 94 year old."[64] Dr. Rowen's father did a complete about-face on selling the machine, and now uses it on many of the health problems he faces.

The improvement in Dr. Rowen's father's cognitive function is consistent with findings from a study on PEMF effects on the brain.[65] The study authors found a 69 percent reduction in ischemic (cut-off blood flow) neuronal damage after treating with PEMF. The treatment was also found helpful for MS, cognitive function, mobility, spasticity, and vision.

The summary of Eastern European research contains an entire section on research into neurological conditions, including MS, cerebrovascular atherosclerosis, atherosclerotic encephalopathy, syringomyelia and post-traumatic cystic myelopathy, peripheral nerve disorders, spinal cord injuries, neuroinfections, and several others.[66] Improvements in these conditions when treated by PEMF ranged from minor to extremely significant. Clearly, PEMF has very hopeful application to pain arising from neurological conditions. If your pain comes from one of these conditions, PEMF would seem to be a very promising therapy for you to try.

NASA has done research on the enhancement of tissue repair in animals. The agency found that PEMF stimulates the generation of stem cells within the body.[67] As most of us have heard in the news over the past several years, stem cells are a subject of intense interest among scientists and researchers. Such cells can become many other types of cells within the body and regenerate prolifically, thus greatly enhancing healing. A technology that causes the body itself to generate new stem cells is thus a huge discovery, and its application is incredibly broad. This may account for the extremely diverse body of research in Eastern Europe. Likewise, it may account for the nearly equally broad realm of efficacious application in a 94-year-old man with the legion of health concerns typical for that stage of life.

PEMF devices vary greatly in their configurations. Some work by creating magnetic fields on mats that you lie on. Others have smaller pads that you place against more targeted sites on your body. Others have probes for precise placement of the magnetic field, and there is at least one machine that uses two ring-shaped field generators that you can place on your body either side by side or on opposing sides of, say, a shoulder or knee, to cause the field to penetrate from one side of the body to the other. The magnetic fields generated by the machines fall off quickly from the point where they're generated, so effective distance from the rings can be extended by placing them on either side of a limb or other portion of the body.

The prices of instruments reflect the limited competition in the field, and are often cost-prohibitive for individuals. The machine with the ring-shaped magnetic field generators described

---

64   How to give your cells a massage and treat impossible-to-cure ailments. *Second Opinion*. 2013;23(1):4.
65   Grant G, Cadossi R, Steinberg G. Protection against focal cerebral ischemia following exposure to a pulsed electromagnetic field. *Bioelectromagnetics*. 1994;15(3):205-216.
66   *Magnetic Therapy in Eastern Europe*; 40-50.
67   Give your cells a massage; 4.

above is one of the lesser-priced models. It's called a SomaPulse, and it costs $1,390. You can read more about the machine or order one at somapulse.com.

The high-end machine Dr. Rowen's father bought was a PMT-100, available at pemf.us. I tried to research this machine and the company behind it, but my experience with the contact person listed on the Web site was less than fully informative. When I asked for information on the company(ies) who did business through the Web site, I was met with silence. I suspect that they are Eastern European companies that want to keep a low profile in the U.S. I asked if he would at least give me a price list for the machines they offer. He did do that. The PMT-100 is offered, at this writing, for $21,000 (ostensibly a $6,000 discount off of retail). Accessory options yield possibilities to purchase the machine for from $20,000 to $23,500. If you are able to afford such a machine, and have myriad health challenges, Dr. Rowen's father's experience suggests this might be the way to go.

For the rest of us, iMRS, at iMRS.com, might have an option that is more within reach. This company offers a rent-to-own option that at this writing costs $500 for one month on a $2,450 machine. The company takes a $1,000 deposit when you rent one of their machines (for a total initial cost of $1,500). If you opt to buy the machine, iMRS applies your rent and deposit toward the purchase (tax and shipping charges apply). If you do not elect to buy the machine, you will pay only the $500 and shipping charges. Your deposit will be returned to you.

This is an excellent chance to see if PEMF will work for your health challenges. Your risk is limited, and you needn't purchase an expensive machine that might not work for you. If it does work for your health issue, you can purchase the machine and use it as extensively as you like forever after. One thing I would advise: If you rent the machine, be sure to experiment with it extensively (within the constraints stipulated by the manufacturer; strong Herxheimer [detox] reactions have been experienced by treating too long at one time with PEMF machines). Many conditions respond to intensity and length of exposure, so experiment freely with it. If you don't experience a quick response to the therapy, you might need to try a different angle; point, length, or frequency of exposure; or type of applicator. The machine is yours for a month. Make good use of it.

A final option is to find a doctor who incorporates a PEMF machine into his practice. I have not found a list of such doctors, but a few of them have independent Web sites you can view. If you search for PEMF on the Internet, some of these sites will show up in your search results. At this writing, there are not many to choose from, but you might be one of the lucky few who have a practitioner nearby. If you don't, the rental option listed above might cost you only a little more than several trips to the doctor's office.

Part 3

Therapies for Joint and Deep-tissue Injuries

Conventional medicine has some ability when it comes to reassembling broken body parts. In regard to helping the healing process, however, it's at a loss. These therapies are not. Many of them greatly speed healing, and some of them promote healing in injuries or conditions where the body has long since done all the healing it intends to do.

Chapter 12

Oxygenation Therapies

In his study "Oxygen in Wound Healing and Infection,"[68] Dr. Finn Gottrup sums up a crucial truth: "It is a fundamental clinical observation that wounds do not heal in tissue that does not bleed, and they almost always heal in tissue that bleeds extensively. Continuous supply of oxygen to the tissue through microcirculation is vital for the healing process and for resistance to infection." He further observes that: "During wound healing, the continuity and function of the damaged tissue are re-established. This is only possible through a restoration of the microcirculation and thereby the nutrition to the tissue. *The main component of the nutrition is oxygen*, which is critically important for healing a wound by production of granulation tissue and for ensuring resistance against infection. This has been shown experimentally, but recently a short period of supplementary oxygen has been shown to decrease wound complications in clinical practice as well." (Emphasis added.)

If a tree falls on your house, you first remove the tree and any damaged portions of the house. Then you cover the exposed area with plastic to keep out the weather and debris, and you "flood the area" with builders and new construction materials to rebuild the broken portions of the house. Your body does things similarly. When it's injured, inflammation immediately begins to isolate and remove infective organisms and materials; it floods the area with blood, while cutting off external bleeding through clotting; and it brings in a rich supply of nutrients to rebuild. But while the materials you'll use to rebuild your house are not living, the materials your body uses are very much alive. They need fuel to do their work. And the most important nutrient living tissues need as they rebuild the damage is oxygen.

Our house analogy is rough, but it works for our purposes. Oxygen's (very rough) counterpart in the analogy is probably the builders, since they animate the process and make it possible. The body provides a certain number of builders when an injury occurs – as many as it can spare. But if you can increase the number of builders, you can greatly accelerate the process. That's what increasing oxygen to the wound does for you. Assuming you have enough other materials for the construction, having more builders will get the job done faster, and probably better.

This enabling of repair and healing is the mechanism of action at the heart of a variety of oxygen therapies, including intravenous hydrogen peroxide (H_2O_2), which breaks down into water (H_2O) and oxygen (O_2) in the body; exercise with oxygen therapy (EWOT), hyperbaric oxygen therapy (HBOT), and even prolozone therapy, which makes use of ozone (O_3) that breaks

68   Gottrup F. Oxygen in wound healing and infection. *World J Surg*. 2004;28(3):312-315. Epub 2004 Feb 17.

down into oxygen in the body. Prolozone, however, will be dealt with in the next chapter along with its progenitor, prolotherapy.

Unlike some therapies (such as massage) that must typically wait for the initial inflammatory period of healing to pass before beginning, oxygen therapies can begin immediately. In fact, the earlier the better. The body's need for increased oxygen to isolate, sterilize, repair, and heal an injury begins immediately, and oxygen is used in each of those processes.

Hydrogen Peroxide Therapy

Intravenous hydrogen peroxide (H_2O_2) therapy is a remarkably versatile treatment with implications for such varied conditions as lung disease, Multiple Sclerosis, Parkinson's, candida, and even periodontal disease (and dozens more). More immediately applicable to the realm of pain, however, it has been used successfully in the treatment of headaches, chronic pain, rheumatoid arthritis, and shingles. It is less often used for wounds or injuries, but I would not hesitate to use it in that capacity. Its broad benefits for bodily tissues and various diseases and conditions indicate its general safety and application to many health issues. In particular, its usefulness in treating diabetic gangrene is strongly indicative of its tissue-healing capabilities. And anyone who has used store-bought H_2O_2 on a cut or abrasion of the skin can readily attest to its healing properties on injured tissue. (The type of H_2O_2 you get at the store is typically 3.5% pharmaceutical grade, which is very different from the H_2O_2 used internally. The former contains several stablizers, such as acetanilide, phenol, sodium stanate, and tertrasodium phosphate, that should not be taken internally.)

Physicians use a very specific protocol, though more than one is in use. They generally add a 30% reagent grade hydrogen peroxide to water, filter it, then add it to a dextrose/water solution. This produces a 0.0375% H_2O_2, 5% dextrose solution that is injected intravenously or intra-arterially. Magnesium is sometimes added to reduce irritation at the injection site. The procedure usually lasts from an hour and a half to two hours. At the practitioner's office, you simply sit in a comfortable chair, allow the practitioner to start an IV drip, and read a book or watch TV for 90 to 120 minutes. It's about as low-stress as it gets.

I'd tell you the mechanism by which H_2O_2 works, but no one fully understands it. Side effects to H_2O_2 therapy are rare, and usually involve irritation of the vein. Much higher concentrations of H_2O_2 used in Europe and elsewhere, while producing generally better results, result in more common and serious injury to veins. Problems in America usually tend to be either irritation at the needle entry site or a red streak up the vein that indicates irritation to a greater extent. Simply moving the needle to another vein usually solves the problem. Another side effect can be temporary shortness of breath, which is not typically significant. Many doctors simply continue the procedure if the problem is not too troubling to the patient. If the patient desires, or the problem is serious enough to concern the practitioner, they either slow the procedure down or stop it altogether.

This lung effect is of unknown cause, but might be related to H_2O_2 therapy's ability to cleanse the lungs of infection and even particulate matter. Patients with significant lung problems often describe the effect as a bubbling up from under the surface of the lungs, carrying mucus and contaminants with it. People with lung issues often start coughing during or shortly after the procedure, trying to expel the contaminants already being lifted from the surface of their lungs.

For information on where to find a practitioner of H_2O_2 therapy, go to the ACAM site at acamnet.org.

The next two oxygen therapies work by getting oxygen into places in the body that typically receive low levels of oxygen, and that, when oxygen flow is decreased, can become oxygen-starved. This especially includes joints and extremities (hands and feet). The first therapy works by inhaling oxygen-enriched air while exercising, and the second works by breathing oxygen in a pressurized chamber – causing oxygen to impregnate the tissues to a much greater degree than normal.

Exercise with Oxygen Therapy (or Oxygen Multistep Therapy)

Exercise with oxygen therapy (EWOT), pioneered by a German scientist, Manfred von Ardenne (who called it oxygen multistep therapy – a name still frequently used today), is the first therapy described above. It entails exercising while breathing from an oxygen concentrator – a device that removes nitrogen from the ambient air and thus delivers approximately 95 percent oxygen through a mask worn over the mouth and nose.

Von Ardenne studied the way the body delivered oxygen to its many destinations at the very ends of the blood delivery system – in the capillaries. He found that capillary flow could be easily disrupted by such things as acute injuries, surgery, or heart attacks. He even found that viral illnesses could reduce flow at this level. The damage done by aging or long-term exposure to toxic chemicals could also reduce capillary blood flow over time. However, the reductions in flow caused by all these injuries proved largely reversible.

His research found that such injuries to the capillaries, whether acute or chronic, cause a tiny ring of muscle that surrounds the arteriole (the smallest vessel for arterial blood flow) to tighten. This impedes blood that is trying to enter the capillaries, which reduces the amount of oxygen getting to bodily tissues. When this phenomenon occurs throughout the body, there are several consequences: many metabolic functions are affected, energy declines, and weakness occurs. But in the presence of increased oxygen, these adverse effects can be reversed. Though the oxygen-carrying capability of each red blood cell is not increased, in the presence of increased oxygen coming into the lungs blood serum levels of oxygen *are* increased. This increase makes the difference.

Von Ardenne therefore developed a technique that today most people call exercise with oxygen therapy. By walking or jogging on a treadmill or pedaling a stationary bicycle while breathing oxygen-intense air, serum oxygen levels are increased enough to deliver a strong therapeutic effect. This can easily be demonstrated in the case of viral infections such as influenza, where 15 minutes to a half-hour of exercise with oxygen can quickly and thoroughly dispel the effects of the infection.

In the case of injury, the same oxygen-enriching effect causes a significantly increased rate of healing, and thus, often, pain relief. Oxygen-rich tissues equate to much better wound or injury healing, provided that adequate nutrients are available for rebuilding from the diet (food and nutritional supplements).

The same effect can be had at a slower rate if you are unable to exercise, but simply breathe oxygen-rich air. Alternatively, if you have an infrared sauna, simply breathe the oxygen while in the sauna. The sauna causes the body to respond in much the same way as exercise, causing more rapid uptake of the oxygen into the tissues. (But heed the previous safety warning about using oxygen in a sauna – there's a potential for an explosion.)

Any way you do it, the oxygen enrichment that comes from this therapy is an important accelerant to the healing process. Studies done in Germany took patients in their 80s and administered EWOT to them. The participants included accident victims, heart attack patients, and people who had had surgery. Each group benefitted from a significant increase in oxygen utilization that lasted for months.

Some EWOT practitioners have observed a strong detoxification effect after treatment. This probably results from the increased cell metabolism that oxygen enrichment makes possible. One of the consequences of this detox phenomenon is that some patients undergo a Herxheimer reaction (nausea and weakness – sometimes severe – caused by the sudden expulsion of too many bio-organisms and/or toxins for the body to handle in an orderly manner). Normally, however, as with many detoxification protocols, this short-term reaction to the cleansing of toxins is followed by an improved sense of well-being.

Hyperbaric Oxygen Therapy

The second of these oxygen enrichment techniques that provides increased oxygen flow to normally hard-to-reach bodily tissues is hyperbaric oxygen therapy (HBOT). This is the treatment given to deep sea divers who surface from ocean depths too quickly and encounter decompression sickness. Essentially, HBOT entails entering a sealed room, pod, or capsule where the air pressure can be increased to about three times normal. Then the person inside the enclosure breathes pure oxygen. In the increased pressure environment, the lungs can absorb about three times as much oxygen as normal. Moreover, the pressure drives oxygen deep into bodily tissues, oxygenating injured tissues in joints that are able to use the increase to repair themselves.

HBOT can't really be termed an alternative treatment anymore. It is in broad use in many mainstream clinics for wound healing due to such things as diabetes, radiation injury, or non-healing wounds. It's also used for carbon monoxide poisoning and bacterial infections such as gas gangrene or bone infections. Professional sports teams also use it to speed the rate of healing in injured players. All of these uses point to the reason HBOT is useful in pain relief – it can cause a rapid increase in the rate of healing in injured or infected tissues.

For this therapy, you will be seated in a small pod or capsule (most clinics use small units, which are more economical than the larger units used in the past to treat divers with the bends). Some of them look a bit like a cockpit from an F-16 without the rest of the plane. Others look like a very large version of the air tube capsule you use in the drive-through section at the bank. The unit will then be slowly pressurized as you are given 100 percent oxygen to breathe. Claustrophobia can be a problem in these small units, though they typically have transparent canopies or windows to reduce this problem. Your ears must also be able to adjust to the pressure changes, so anything that prevents doing so (such as a sinus infection) could delay you from undergoing the therapy. A few patients have changes in vision related to the pressure, but these typically resolve within eight weeks of the therapy. Keep in mind that three atmospheres of pressure, which is typically the high end in these hyperbaric oxygen units (lower pressures are often used), is equivalent to scuba diving at a depth of 66 feet. That is not a shallow dive, but it is not a particularly deep one, either.

Each treatment will last from an hour and 15 minutes to an hour and a half. You can typically read a book or watch TV while you undergo the treatment, so it's pretty low-stress. Once you adjust to the higher pressure by using a Valsalva maneuver (closing the mouth, pinching the nostrils shut, and trying to blow to equalize the pressure in the ears) or swallowing, you probably won't feel a thing. Your ears will likely adjust to the lessening of pressure at the end of the treatment without any help.

In addition to wound and injury healing, HBOT has been used for fibromyalgia, rheumatoid arthritis, Buerger's disease, burns, and many other conditions.[69] Contrary to what you might suspect if you've read too much about oxidation/free radical creation, oxygenation of tissues is typically a very, very good thing.[70] While conventional medicine is quick to point out that scientific studies are lacking for many of these applications, practitioners are equally quick to point out that HBOT often works when other modalities do not. It's your choice: acceptance or efficacy. There are times when you can't have both.

If you have an injury, wound, nerve condition, recent surgery, degenerative disease, or headache, give one of these oxygen therapies a try. All three have extremely wide application to

---

69   Elmer M. Cranton, M.D. offers a fairly comprehensive list at http://drcranton.com/hbo/conditions_treated.htm.
70   Free radicals are necessary for good health. The body's immune system often creates them to battle bacteria and viruses. It's only when the body does not have enough antioxidants to neutralize them that they get out of control and do serious damage.

a variety of conditions, and chances are you'll experience some welcome relief. All three tend to have cumulative effects, meaning that several treatments are better than one or two. But all have an enviable track record of restoring health to many suffering patients.

Locate a practitioner as near you as possible and give them a call. (Lack of mainstream acceptance means practitioners must usually set up shop near a major population center, which means travel for many of us.) ACAM lists practitioners at acamnet.org. Ask if it's worthwhile to try their specialty on your particular source of pain. If their answer is satisfying and their price is right, give it a try.

Chapter 13

Prolotherapies

The prolotherapies are particularly potent tools in the pain relief kit. In the very big world of joint injuries, there are few, if any, tools as capable of healing old (often very old) injuries. Oxygen therapies are immensely helpful in aiding the healing process right after injury, and also have application to injuries after the passage of time. But the prolotherapies concentrate healing processes directly in the joint, and are therefore more intense and more specifically efficacious.

There are basically two kinds of prolotherapy, though there are variations within each kind. The first, both in chronology and number of practitioners, is prolotherapy itself. The term prolotherapy is short for proliferation therapy, which gives some clue as to its mechanism of action. It is basically geared at instigating an inflammatory response at the injured site, which causes blood vessels to proliferate, thus stimulating healing.

Prolozone, in contrast, contains an oxygen/ozone mix that doesn't rely on stimulating your body to supply blood, and thus oxygen, to the injured site. It supplies the oxygen directly. As a result, it can often prompt very rapid rates of healing in oxygen-poor joint tissues.

Prolotherapy

Prolotherapy originated in 1937 when a surgeon named Dr. Earl Gedney caught his thumb in the doors to his operating room and stretched the tendons, causing great pain and instability. He was told that there was no help for his condition, and that his operating career was over.

Rather than submit to such a dire prognosis, however, he started doing some research. He found that doctors who were dealing with hernia treatments had developed an innovative technique. It involved strengthening the tissue surrounding a hernia by injecting an irritant solution into the tissue. He adapted this concept and used it to heal his hand. His success was so complete that he was able to restore his hand to full use.

Prolotherapy has made a number of appearances in the scientific literature between then and now, but it has never made it into mainstream medicine. It remains, however, one of the most powerful modalities in existence for actually healing injured joints. Surgery can do much to put tissues back in their proper place, but it can do little to speed the healing process inherent in the body. It basically resets the joint in as close to original condition as possible and lets the body's inherent healing processes take over.

In contrast, prolotherapy greatly speeds those processes. In the original and most common form of this treatment, a solution is injected near or into the joint that is causing problems. The solution often contains a mild sugar, such as hyperosmolar dextrose, or salt, with the pain-killer lidocaine. Other solutions are also used. These solutions are mildly irritating to the tissues surrounding the joint, and this irritation causes a low-grade inflammatory response from the body. As far as the body is concerned, an injury has recurred at the site, so the body kicks into repair mode, growing new blood vessels into the area and flooding it with nutrients and oxygen to rebuild injured tissue. By repeatedly injecting the site, the perception of injury can be maintained and the healing response greatly lengthened and heightened.

This is necessary because the healing process in blood-poor joints is typically insufficient to restore 100 percent functionality, flexibility, and strength. Most of the healing response occurs in the first week after injury, and most of the healing is complete within the first month. Though healing continues thereafter, it does so at a low and ever-declining rate. Because less (often *much* less) than 100 percent of functionality is restored, the joint is susceptible to further injury, which further reduces functionality, and the cycle can continue indefinitely. By greatly extending and enriching the healing process, functionality can often be fully restored. Many patients report a return of joint strength and mobility superior to that which they enjoyed prior to the injury.

The issue of tissue proximity that allows prolotherapy to be efficacious is, in another respect, also a major part of what prolotherapy provides. By that I mean that many joint injuries are either caused by or result in stretched ligaments. And prolotherapy can cause these ligaments to tighten, which pulls the joint into alignment and strengthens it.

Ligaments are strong, fibrous tissues that connect bones to other bones in a joint (in contrast, tendons connect muscles to bones). If you were to see beneath the skin of your body, you would see that your muscles are red, while your tendons and ligaments are white. The reason for this, as Donna Alderman, D.O., illustrates in her excellent book *Free Yourself from Chronic Pain and Sports Injuries* (an excellent book about prolotherapy), is that there is little blood in tendons and ligaments.[71]

As you age, the cartilage in your joints wears away or is compacted. Cartilage is a very tough, rubber-like tissue (also white and blood-poor) that cushions and lubricates the space between bones within the joints. Activity, impact, injury, and chronic inflammation can cause the gradual thinning and even virtual disappearance of this layer of cartilage. As that happens, the ligaments that stretch over the gap between the bones, joining those bones tightly when the cartilage buffer is at full depth, tend to become loose. The loss of cartilage causes the bones to move closer together, and their connecting ligaments do not tighten to adjust for the change.

This phenomenon is so important that it likely explains not only an effect from injury, but a major *cause* of injury. Loose ligaments probably precede many injuries, allowing them to happen because the joint is no longer tight and strong. This is likely a major cause of lower back injuries,

---

71   2008, Family Doctor Press, pp12-13.

where cartilage is subject to especially strong impact and compressive forces, and in many people begins compacting at a relatively young age. The resulting looseness in the ligaments that connect the lumbar vertebrae allows a simple act such as bending at the waist to rupture a disk. The joint is not held tightly together by the ligaments, and simple leverage takes over when the vertebrae bend at an improper angle to one another and highly stress the cartilaginous disk, thus rupturing it.

Some doctors feel that this sequence of events is also a major cause of osteoarthritis. When an injury occurs, the movement in the joint changes. Suboptimal stresses are induced. Bone responds to stress by adding more bone, which can increase bone-on-bone contact, friction, and stress. Or it can cause the bone to impinge on soft tissue. Either way, it causes stress, an inflammatory response, and ultimately arthritis.[72]

So either damaged cartilage or a stretched ligament can be a precursor to arthritis by creating laxity in the joint. Importantly, however, a loose ligament does not prompt an adequate healing response by the body. It will remain loose indefinitely unless such a healing response is initiated. When mild inflammation is triggered by prolotherapy, it activates fibroblasts (cells that help form connective tissue) in the area. These help develop collagen, which is a very strong protein the body uses in many connective tissues, such as skin, ligaments, tendons, and bone. Loss of collagen or an insufficient amount of it causes looseness, weakness, and/or a loss of elasticity in the affected tissue.

Through this means, prolotherapy strongly promotes collagen growth in loose or injured tissues, thus restoring strength, flexibility, and functionality to injured or unstable joints. This can actually prevent osteoarthritis from developing because it prevents chronic inflammation. If arthritis is already present, it can often stimulate enough healing in the soft tissues of the joint to relieve the pain. One study found that "though the osteoarthritis that has developed does not go away, a remarkable thing has been observed in many people with osteoarthritis after prolotherapy – the *pain* reduces or goes away."[73]

Prolotherapy is very, very useful medicine, and it has the capability to completely restore many dysfunctional joints and stop or greatly alleviate the associated pain. Many thousands of people have undergone prolotherapy and experienced amazing healing. And while there is some good science on this (several studies have been done), it is still avoided and panned by conventional medicine. However, some of the anecdotes available will amaze you. Dr. Alderman includes many detailed testimonials in her book, together with full names and quite a bit of detail. Some of my friends and associates have given me similar accounts. And because we're talking here about major structural healing, the placebo effect is not a very satisfying explanation for the multitude of people who report real, substantial relief. Prolotherapy is clearly something you

---

72 *Free Yourself from Chronic Pain,* 111-114.
73 Reeves KD, Hassanein K. Randomized prospective double-blind placebo-controlled study of dextrose prolotherapy for knee osteoarthritis with or without ACL laxity. *Alternative Therapies.* 2000;6:68-80.

should look into if your pain comes from a joint injury or problem.

Traditional prolotherapy is not your only option, however. Two other forms of prolotherapy have also arisen in recent years. Platelet rich plasma, or PRP, therapy is one of the new forms, and biocellular prolotherapy is the other. Each offers important new capabilities to the process of injecting healing-promoting substances into injured tissues.

PRP therapy involves enriching a quantity of the patient's own withdrawn blood to the point where, instead of a normal six percent platelets, it contains 94 percent platelets. Platelets are so called because under the microscope they look like little plates. They are produced in the bone marrow and circulate freely in the blood. When you suffer a cut in your skin, they are responsible for clotting the blood and starting the healing process in the wound. PRP contains seven growth factors that cause this healing to begin. It is rich with repair cells and stem cells that kick healing into overdrive.

The process was used in the early 2000s as an aid to bone grafts and fractures, and later was used in sports medicine for connective tissue repair. Athletes such as Pittsburgh Steelers' wide receiver Hines Ward, LA Dodgers' closing pitcher Takashi Saito, and golfer Tiger Woods publicly credited PRP for helping them return to their respective sports after significant injuries. PRP is in increasing use for the treatment of such problems as ligament and tendon injuries, osteoarthritis, degenerative cartilage, chronic elbow tendonosis, muscle strain and tears, plantar fasciitis, and rotator cuff tendinopathy.[74]

A study was published in the January 13, 2010, issue of the *Journal of the American Medical Association*, comparing PRP therapy with saline (i.e. salt water) injection (essentially saline prolotherapy) in the treatment of chronic achilles tendinopathy.[75] The study's authors found essentially no difference in outcome between the two modalities, though both were found to offer "significant" improvement in the subjects studied. Clearly, there is a good bit of overlap between the two therapies, but there may be cases where PRP is preferred: "When PRP is used as a prolotherapy 'formula' for chronic or longstanding injuries, the PRP increases the initial healing factors and thereby the rate of healing."[76]

Biocellular prolotherapy is yet another modality that involves the proliferation of healing mechanisms at an injury site. In this case, however, the cells that provide the healing are not necessarily indigenous cells to the injury site, but cells injected from elsewhere in the patient's body. The reason this can be necessary is that a very old, unhealed injury might have exhausted the healing capacity of the cells around it. This is called "cellular depletion," and bodes ill for therapies geared to stimulating the body's own healing capabilities. Dextrose prolotherapy, PRP,

74   Platelet rich plasma therapy. prolotherapy.com/PlateletRichPlasmaProlotherapy.php. Accessed September 4, 2013.
75   de Vos RJ, Weir A, van Schie HTM, Bierma-Zeinstra SMA, Verhaar JAN, Weinans H, Tol JL. Platelet-rich plasma injection for chronic Achilles tendinopathy. *JAMA*. 2010;303(2):144-149. doi:10.1001/jama.2009.1986.
76   Platelet rich plasma therapy. prolotherapy.com/PlateletRichPlasmaProlotherapy.php. Accessed September 4, 2013.

and even prolozone (to be discussed in the next section) fall into that category, so biocellular prolotherapy can be a much-needed adjunct to the prolotherapist's medical bag.

If prolotherapy sounds like a promising therapy for your type of pain, talk to a doctor who's knowledgeable about your particular injury and the various options to treat it. Dr. Alderman is certainly one such doctor, having learned her craft from some of the pioneers in the field, but there are many others throughout the country. Try to talk to several doctors, ask if you can talk to some of their patients (or better yet, find patients through your personal network or via the Internet), and ask the doctors what kind of success they've enjoyed. Dr. William Campbell Douglass recommends that you ask if they have ever been *successfully* sued for malpractice. Despite all the frivolous suits filed in America, he notes that those who are actually sued successfully (not just sued – that can happen to anyone) are often guilty of sloppy or incompetent medical practice. In short: In this field, as in every other, there are people who know what they're doing and others who are basically "me, too" practitioners. You definitely want one of the former.

Prolozone

As useful and efficacious as prolotherapy is, one doctor grew frustrated with the time (and associated expense) that it sometimes entailed. He understood the mechanism by which it healed, but he wondered if that mechanism's effects could be attained via a quicker route. Essentially, prolotherapy works because it causes the body to build new supply routes (blood vessels) to the injury site, which provide nutrients and oxygen to the injured area. Dr. Frank Shallenberger wondered if there was a way to provide the most essential of the rebuilding nutrients – oxygen – to the injury quickly, without necessarily having to prompt the body to provide it.

His experimentation eventually led him to begin using a mixture of oxygen (O_2) and ozone (O_3) that he injects into the tissue surrounding an injury. The oxygen has immediate application because it is obviously what the tissues need to conduct the healing process, but why ozone?

There are a number of reasons. According to one of the Web sites Dr. Shallenberger is associated with,[77] these are a few of ozone's benefits:

1. **Ozone is anti-aging.** Some of those anti-aging effects can be attributed to the following factors in this list.

2. **Ozone increases oxygenation of your cells** (it has been proven that cancer and disease grow in poorly oxygenated tissues in your body).

3. **Ozone modulates your immune system.** (For those with a weakened immune system, ozone will boost the immune system. For those with auto-immune disorders, ozone will modulate the immune system to help to stop it from attacking healthy human cells.)

---

77 **Ozone therapy information, ozone therapy articles, and ozone therapy studies.** "Oxygen Healing Thera-pies." oxygenhealingtherapies.com/ozone_therapy.html. Accessed August 24, 2013.

4. **Ozone increases energy production in your cells.** (Your cells need energy to be healthy; low energy levels mean that *you* and *your cells* will not be healthy and will age.)

5. **Ozone increases the activity of your "anti-oxidant enzyme systems."** This means ozone will *reduce* the oxidation levels of your body.

6. **Ozone reduces the level of acidity of your body.** (Never mind drinking alkaline water, you can achieve the same effect with ozone!)

7. **Ozone kills bacteria and viruses** (and virtually all other disease-causing organisms) on contact.

8. **Ozone kills cancer cells on contact.**

When you go in to get prolozone, the doctor will prepare some large syringes with an oxygen/ozone solution in them. Depending on the doctor, a preinjection may be used that contains vitamins, minerals, and homeopathics. In my case, injections were made on either side of my spine in the lower back and in the back of my shoulder. It feels like the area gets very full, which in effect it does as the gas goes into the tissue. It's not pleasant, but it's not unbearable, either.

The oxygen/ozone mix immediately begins to suffuse through the tissues in the vicinity of the injection site. Cells that badly want to go into healing action are finally able to do so because of the oxygen they receive. Oxygen is the key. Once it's there, the healing process starts moving again. The cells can begin to repair themselves and the tissues around them, and they can excrete waste materials and function as they should.

The ozone mix stimulates cellular growth factors, including growth factor beta (TGF-B). This cytokine causes cartilage cells to produce the proteins needed for the production of cartilage. X-ray evidence shows that prolozone can actually cause the regeneration of cartilage. It causes tissue regeneration and the buildup of antioxidant enzymes, and it reduces inflammation. Few other therapies can boast such powerful healing effects.

The therapy's inventor reports his patients typically experience a 70 percent complete healing rate when treated with this therapy. And he states that the other 30 percent of his patients are substantially helped by it.

Having undergone treatment from Dr. Shallenberger and a couple of the doctors he has trained, I can say that this is the most effective treatment I have undergone for my back. It gave me back some of the strength and flexibility I had lost for decades, and relieved much of my pain. Even at that, I was clearly in the 30 percent, not the 70 percent. Don't be discouraged by that, however, as my back injury is a very serious one, and my MRI shows some significant structural damage. If prolozone can help such an injury, it is truly a highly effective treatment.

Prolozone typically heals much more quickly, and with far fewer injections, than traditional prolotherapy. Back when he primarily used prolotherapy, Dr. Shallenberger typically needed 10 to 20 injections to attain success. With prolozone, he typically needs only three to six. He likens a prolotherapy injection to a rifle shot – it's very effective, but you really need to hit what you're aiming at. Prolozone, however, is more like a shotgun blast. You just need to get it in the vicinity and it will do the job.

That was certainly my experience, with one exception. Dr. Shallenberger used prolozone on my injured left knee, but was not able to get the solution in the right place. The physiology of my knee is altered enough, and the scar tissue is so extensive, that the normal injection site wasn't appropriate for me. Accordingly, I experienced no benefit from that particular injection. So although this therapy has a broad-area effect, there are certain physiological barriers that can significantly block or impede its work. When such barriers are not present, the shotgun effect he describes is accurate. Prolozone completely healed a severe shoulder injury for me within five injections, though tissues throughout the shoulder had been badly torn.[78]

Dr. Shallenberger has also found prolozone effective in treating rheumatoid arthritis-induced swelling, pain, and dysfunction in joints. As he was developing the technique, one lady with severe arthritis in her knees asked him to administer prolozone to her. He was doubtful that it would work as well as with injuries, but the effect was strong and positive. Additionally, Dr. Rowen has treated many patients with severe arthritis. Many of them have experienced almost total remission of the pain and swelling they earlier suffered from.

In short, when it comes to serious joint injuries or arthritis pain and inflammation, prolozone is one of the most efficacious therapies available. For the many severe joint injuries I've experienced, it has been by far the most effective therapy I've come across. My case may not be typical (I suspect many people actually have significantly better results than mine, as did my brother, though one acquaintance of mine was not helped by the one injection she was able to undergo), but the many successes experienced by Drs. Rowen and Shallenberger, along with their many colleagues, attest that the therapy has amazing capabilities to heal.

Dr. Shallenberger has trained many other doctors in the administration of prolozone. You can find out if there's one near you by going to oxygenhealingtherapies.com/ and clicking on the little purple button on the left side of the page labeled "Ozone Doctors." That will take you to a page where you just click on your state, province, or country to find out who's practicing in your vicinity. Not every doctor listed offers prolozone, but if they do it will be noted.

The American Academy of Ozonotherapy also maintains a doctor-search function on its site, aaot.us. Just click on the button labeled "Find a Doctor" and look for doctors with "APT" annotated after their names. This indicates that they have undergone prolozone training.

---

78   Shallenberger F. Do away with shoulder pain permanently – no surgery required. *Real Cures*, 2009;8(1):2.

Chapter 14

Manipulation Therapies

Physical manipulation of the body is capable of far greater therapeutic effects than are typically recognized by either conventional medicine or modern people in general. Its efficacy is likely due to two main factors. First, humans need the touch of other people. This has long been recognized in child development, but it's true in adults, as well. A study on the importance of touch for healthy childhood development also recognized that employees who were afforded seated massages at work were healthier, less stressed, and more productive. Of children it said: "orphaned infants exposed to the bleakest of conditions in eastern European institutions exhibited impaired growth and cognitive development, as well as an elevated incidence of serious infections…."[79] The health effects of touch are clearly quite significant.

But second, the human ability to manipulate things is extraordinary. This is not only due to the dexterity of the human hand and the presence of an opposing thumb, though these are key things. It is also due to the clarity and depth of vision the human eye affords and the complexity of thought the human brain is capable of. Thus, while anthropologists might go all weak in the knees over a chimpanzee using a rock to break open a nut, humans can paint a Rembrandt, compose and play a Beethoven symphony, sculpt a David, write and perform Romeo and Juliet, build an Empire State Building or an Apollo rocket, and much, much more. And they can certainly use their brains, eyes, and hands to explore, diagnose, and treat abnormalities in human physiology. This capability has limits, of course, but it has *far* greater scope than most people suspect.

In this section, we'll look at some of these amazing techniques of manual manipulation of the body. Remarkable strides have been made in these disciplines. We don't always know why they work, but, given the elementary and very direct way in which the therapies are applied, the evidence of their efficacy is often immediate and clear. And even when they take some time to have full effect, their results are tangible and unmistakable. With that introduction, let's examine some of these wonderful therapies.

Osteopathic Manipulation

The osteopathic physician is in a position to be the most complete and well-rounded physician possible. That's because he or she is trained in all aspects of medical treatment

---

79 Ardiel EL and Rankin CH. The importance of touch in development. *Paediatr Child Health.* 2010;15(3):153–156.

in which the M.D. is trained, plus some others. I'm referring here to both the philosophy of osteopathy, which is holistic and emphasizes analysis and treatment of the body as an integrated whole rather than a collection of parts and systems, and the specific training in treatment of the musculoskeletal elements of the body. Manipulation of the body is a powerful therapeutic tool, and it is missing from the toolbox of most medical doctors.

I was introduced to this power of manipulation about 16 years ago when I visited an osteopathic physician in Denver. At that time, I had lived with my back injury for nearly 17 years, but had not been to an osteopath or chiropractor. That's because I had visited a chiropractor as a child with my mom, but had not benefited from manipulation at that time. I'm not sure why, but I suspect such factors as the nature of my pain, the abilities of the particular doctor, or perhaps the state of chiropractic treatment in that era.

During the course of my office visit in Denver, the doctor asked me to bend forward and come as close as I could to touching the floor. I did so, and came about 15 inches from the floor with my fingertips. He then had me sit on a bench while he felt my spine through the skin of my back. While I was sitting there, he placed his thumb beside one of my vertebrae and pushed. It was a firm push, but nothing drastic. My vertebra moved, he asked me to stand up and repeat my attempt to touch the floor, and I was able to come about an inch from the floor – with no pain. I had not been able to do anything remotely like that since before my injury many years prior. It was an amazing demonstration of knowledge of human anatomy and function, and of skill at restoring the latter.

It's probably true that the doctor I've described is a standout in his field, but I must say that most of the osteopaths I've gone to have been quite good. Unfortunately, though the job description for osteopaths is superior to that for medical doctors, societal approval is lavished on the M.D. far more than on the D.O. Physical manipulation of the body yields no profit for the medical-industrial complex, so M.D.s are the ones the complex put its money and approval behind. Consequently, many of the students whom society regards as the best and brightest head for the medical schools, where far more extensive resources await them (though exceptions abound in both M.D. and D.O. schools).

Just for the record, I have known a number of excellent medical doctors in my time. Some of them transcend their training and become excellent healers. The problem is that they must transcend their training. M.D. training is rigorous, extensive, thorough, and often efficacious – and it has gaps big enough to drive the health of a nation through. Unfortunately, few medical doctors are aware of the vast amount of knowledge they *don't* know. Until relatively recently, nutrition wasn't even taught at all in medical education. It's still not typically taught beyond some cursory basics. That's unbelievable. But med school is esoteric, difficult, and expensive enough to instill enormous pride in its adherents. And pride is much of the problem. Whether you view it proverbially and say that it goes before a fall, or whether you view it practically and say that a proud person isn't sufficiently on the lookout for things that can go wrong or things that can be done differently, the result is the same. It's trouble, and patients often pay the price – both literally and figuratively. As Agatha Christie's Hercule Poirot poignantly noted, "A doctor who lacks doubt is not a doctor. He is an executioner."[80]

With all that said, and getting back to osteopathy, there are many superb osteopathic physicians in practice in America. They typically go into osteopathy out of conviction rather than a desire for prestige, societal acceptance, or outlandish remuneration. And by dint of their training and their post-doctoral self-education, they often offer a truly impressive array of therapeutic options. They understand that many injuries that will heal on their own will heal better if everything is properly aligned. That's huge. Medical doctors will align a broken bone before splinting it, but they do not align a misaligned vertebra before advising a patient that a back injury will likely heal on its own. I know, as I saw several M.D.s after injuring my back. None of them did a thing about alignment. I'm left to wonder how much better my back would function now if I hadn't gone nearly two decades with a badly misaligned vertebra (it could have become misaligned over time, but I'll never know; it wasn't adequately checked at the time of the injury).

When I have a joint injury now, I go to an osteopathic physician. There are two reasons for this. First, as mentioned earlier, they are concerned about the injury in the context of the rest of my body.

Second, because of their "second-class citizen" status as far as society is concerned, a D.O. is more open to viewing medical options on their merits rather than on their acceptability within the conventional medical community. D.O.s are also open to such options because of the holistic emphasis of their education – and frequently their overall way of thinking. This is crucial, and many of the doctors who offer the treatments described in this report are osteopathic physicians. In effect, to some extent, they *live* outside the box, so thinking outside it is natural.

An osteopathic physician can diagnose and treat any disease or injury an M.D. can, but D.O.s tend to be more reluctant to prescribe drugs than are M.D.s. An osteopath will certainly do so if drugs are called for, but the reluctance is refreshing to me. Drugs are far too easily resorted to by most people, both patients and doctors.

If your doctor does not offer a treatment you read about in this report, and is not willing to learn about it, you might try your local osteopathic physician. Even if he or she does not currently offer it, they might be willing to learn the treatment and offer it in the future. I am currently trying to get my osteopathic physician to learn prolozone. He's not there yet, but I'm still working on him.

One final note on osteopathic physicians: D.O.s make great family physicians because of the breadth and depth of their training. In my town, every general practitioner has a long waiting list for new patients. I was instantly able to get an appointment with my D.O., and he's a good doctor. It's something to consider.

80 *Agatha Christie: Poirot,* "The Cornish Mystery."

Chiropractic manipulation

Chiropractic practice has now diversified into so many disciplines that it's impossible to cover them all in this report. Suffice it to say that there are many, many options to try if you're in pain that comes from joint injury. If you don't get relief from one chiropractor, try another. They vary extensively in their abilities and their techniques. I've experienced everything from no relief at all in my childhood to virtually complete relief in recent years.

Here, as with light therapy, you'll experience some modalities that might make you uncomfortable. They're not necessarily based on spiritual precepts, but they're a bit strange in operation. They tend to cause extreme skepticism in people unacquainted with them or the rationale behind them. I'm speaking primarily here about Applied Kinesiology. It involves muscle testing by the doctor, who tells you to hold a limb in a given position while he tries to move it. This tells him whether or not a given limb or your back is properly aligned for optimal function, or whether certain muscles are functioning as they ought. Based on his findings, he'll then adjust you accordingly. When you see it for the first time, you might think it's silly or just plain weird, and you might wonder how it could possibly work, or be of any help.

Frankly, however, it has been the basis for the best chiropractic treatment I've received. Until he retired a couple of years ago, my former chiropractor used kinesiology as his primary treatment method. As truly as I can tell you, he was simply amazing. In the 20 or so visits I made to his office, only once did he fail to give me relief from my back pain that was extensive and thorough (though obviously temporary, typically lasting from several weeks to several months). I told him about the failure when it happened, and he had me come back for a follow-up treatment at no cost, which perfectly relieved my pain.

Many chiropractors now incorporate therapeutic lasers into their practices. Some incorporate other treatments, such as other forms of light therapy or PEMF. Chiropractic treatments are now so popular that competition causes a great deal of innovation and investment in learning the latest information and techniques. The consequence is that many people have experience with chiropractors, and are willing to tell you which doctors are excellent and which are not. Choose one who knows his business, and you'll have an efficacious means of addressing your joint-related pain without the high cost of a medical doctor visit.

I'll take no further time to tell you in this report what you can easily find in far greater depth online, but chiropractic therapy is for real. It has come far from its origins, which were not always as empirically grounded as might be desired, and has become a highly efficacious means of treating pain and dysfunction. A good chiropractor will take your case very personally, and will try a number of modalities to help you feel better and recover from your injury quickly and thoroughly. Mine lent me his bicycle trainer to help me with my latest bout of severe back pain. It helped immensely, and saved me a couple hundred dollars to buy one.

One note of caution here: Chiropractors, like all health professionals (and all people) vary greatly in their competence and in the methods they use. Try hard to get recommendations from people who have gone to several chiropractors. Find out which one has a good reputation. Start there. It can save you a lot of time and money, and address your pain sooner and much more completely. Try chiropractors who use different techniques, as well. Most of the friends who recommended chiropractors to me tried to steer me away from Kinesiology. Fortunately, I tried it anyway and had better results with it than anything else.

Zero Balancing

Zero balancing is another powerful technique that entails skilled use of the hands to restore normalcy to the body. Its mechanism is not understood, and it is another therapy whose practitioners often use energy flow as a goal and proffered mechanism of action. My concerns on that front have been thoroughly presented elsewhere, but Judith Sullivan, a zero balancing practitioner in Virginia, equates energy flow to movement of the body for those of us who have questions about the energy concept. That's a bit easier concept to get one's arms around.

The therapy uses the hands to provide a fulcrum (a fulcrum is similar in function to the pole that a teeter-totter pivots on) for various parts of the body. A skilled practitioner can determine, when placing the fingers at a specific point, whether the muscles or body parts beside the fulcrum (the fingers) are operating properly. Often they are not. By placing gentle pressure on this fulcrum point, the originator of the process, Fritz Frederick Smith, M.D., found that the inoperative muscles were often activated and began working properly. No one has been able to authoritatively explain why this happens, but it's a palpable effect for the practitioner. He or she can feel the muscle or body part begin to function in response to pressure on the fulcrum point.

Though muscles may be the parts of the body that need to be re-started, so to speak, the therapy actually focuses on bones and ligaments. Thus, the fulcrum point is often at a joint. And the therapy also makes use of traction, as in selectively pulling on a limb, to restore movement and normalcy to the body. A patient will therefore typically lie on a table while the practitioner perhaps pulls on one leg or both of them to restore alignment, then works on the hips, ribs, and head using the fulcrum concept. In a session, for example, Ms. Sullivan feels each rib to determine which of them are responsive. If one of them is not (a practitioner will describe them as being "stuck"), she applies gentle pressure to restore its proper movement.

Because parts of the body can so easily get out of proper alignment and either stop working entirely or stop working optimally, restoring proper function has very wide application. Stress-induced problems can be addressed, which in turn tend to reduce the stress that caused them. Back and neck pain; shoulder, knee, and hip pain; temporomandibular joint (jaw) pain; headaches; and many other sources of pain often experience significant or total relief. Ms. Sullivan's Web site lists many other conditions she often treats as well.[81]

---

81 Chijude.com. Accessed September 2, 2013.

Three to four sessions are the average of what's needed for people who see Ms. Sullivan for treatment, typically once per week. At the upper end of skill level and cost, she charges $125 for a 45-minute session. However, a session with her offers patients all of her therapeutic modalities, including craniosacral therapy, which I discuss in the following section. Ms. Sullivan is one of the top people in these disciplines, and many other practitioners charge considerably less.

Craniosacral Therapy

This therapy was developed by an osteopathic physician named John Upledger, with whom Ms. Sullivan studied. During a neck surgery in which Dr. Upledger was assisting, he noticed a rhythmic movement in what he would eventually know as the craniosacral system. This system is defined by Mosby's Dictionary of Complementary and Alternative Medicine as the "physiologic system of cerebrospinal fluid and the dura mater membrane [a thick membrane surrounding the brain, inside the skull] as well as attached bones, sutures, and vessels."[82] The rhythmic phenomenon Dr. Upledger observed was largely unexplored, however, so he had to do quite a bit of research to determine its nature and significance.

The therapy he subsequently developed depended in part on placing very light pressure on various points in the craniosacral system. The pressure used is typically no more than five grams – about the weight of a nickel. This pressure releases restrictions in the soft tissues around the central nervous system, which helps improve resistance to disease, according to practitioners. It also relieves many kinds of pain and dysfunction, some of which are listed below.[83]

- Migraines and Headaches

- Chronic Neck and Back Pain

- Stress and Tension-Related Disorders

- Brain and Spinal Cord Injuries

- Fibromyalgia

- TMJ Syndrome

- Scoliosis

- Central Nervous System Disorders

- Orthopedic Problems

- And Many Other Conditions

---

82   Accessed online on September 2, 2013 at http://medical-dictionary.thefreedictionary.com/craniosacral+system.
83   Frequently Asked Questions – CranioSacral Therapy, Upledger Institute International, upledger.com/content. asp?id=61, accessed September 2, 2013.

Craniosacral therapy posits a controversial claim – that the bones of the skull move in relation to one another. Like any other bones and joints in the body, when these bones become misaligned, they create problems. Realigning them, or removing the tension from them, can be highly therapeutic. Likewise, other misalignments or restrictions in the craniosacral system can be set right, with significant beneficial effects.

To describe the way craniosacral therapy works, the Upledger Institute's description is hard to improve on:

> "Few structures have as much influence over the body's ability to function properly as the brain and spinal cord that make up the central nervous system. And the central nervous system is heavily influenced by the craniosacral system – the membranes and fluid that surround, protect, and nourish the brain and spinal cord.

> "Every day your body endures stresses and strains that it must work to compensate for. Unfortunately, these changes often cause body tissues to tighten and distort the craniosacral system. These distortions can then cause tension to form around the brain and spinal cord resulting in restrictions. This can create a barrier to the healthy performance of the central nervous system, and potentially every other system it interacts with.

> "Fortunately, such restrictions can be detected and corrected using simple methods of touch. With a light touch, the CST practitioner uses his or her hands to evaluate the craniosacral system by gently feeling various locations of the body to test for the ease of motion and rhythm of the cerebrospinal fluid pulsing around the brain and spinal cord. Soft-touch techniques are then used to release restrictions in any tissues influencing the craniosacral system.

> "By normalizing the environment around the brain and spinal cord and enhancing the body's ability to self-correct, CranioSacral Therapy is able to alleviate a wide variety of dysfunctions, from chronic pain and sports injuries to stroke and neurological impairment."[84]

Both zero balancing and craniosacral therapy were recommended to me by my publisher. He suggested I look into them because he had experienced extremely positive results over the course of several years from Ms. Sullivan's treatments. She, in turn, referenced many patients who have had amazing turnarounds in their conditions as a result of one or both of these therapies. Her office charges for craniosacral therapy are the same as for zero balancing, as she uses either or both as a patient's needs may dictate.

Clearly, as with other body-manipulation techniques mentioned in this report, these therapies are highly therapeutic in treating a myriad of health conditions. If craniosacral therapy

---

84   Upledger Institute, Frequently Asked Questions.

or zero balancing is of interest to you, you can find a practitioner near you by going to the International Association of Health Practitioners. Just go to iahp.com and click on the prominent "Search for a Practitioner" button.

Bowen Therapy

Another manipulative technique that employs a very light touch is Bowen Therapy. Unlike zero balancing and craniosacral therapy, Bowen therapy works on muscles.

This is a therapy that has been demonstrated at several doctor conferences in order to make doctors aware of it. Between the doctors who have participated and those who have looked on, quite a number of written testimonies have been published. The testimonials have been almost surreal. Doctor after doctor went up to the front of the assembly, received treatment, and experienced almost instantaneous results. They not only had an almost instant release of pain (which can be subjective), but an equally impressive increase in their range of movement.

Here's what the therapy consists of:

The adjustment of Bowen therapy is called a "move," which is made across or perpendicular to the muscle or tendon, 90 degrees to its line of fibers. The therapist simply places his/her fingers over the central portion of the muscle belly and then stretches the skin across the muscle to contact its edge. Slight pressure is placed on the edge of the muscle belly (in a 90-degree direction to its line of force) so that the muscle is exposed to a gentle perpendicular stretch. Then on the outgoing breath, the practitioner "moves" his fingers across the muscle to the other edge. This results in discharge of the nerve spindles within the muscle or tendon that can cause instant relaxation of that muscle or other associated muscles.

In Bowen therapy, muscle moves apparently have the ability to reset the autonomic nervous system [ANS]. This can result in greater blood flow, oxygen delivery, and restoration of cellular activity in the whole distribution of that segment of the ANS (both in muscles and organs). An added benefit is the stimulation of lymph flow, which aids in detoxification and, thus, cancer prevention.[85]

It's useful in treating many musculoskeletal sources of pain, as well as migraines and other headaches, and a large number of other health challenges. This of course includes many of the most common sources of pain, such as neck, shoulder, arm, back, hip, and knee pain. It has virtually no risks. Usually a patient needs only a few sessions, and they're typically scheduled a week apart.

It's hard to see how this therapy could have any downside other than the cost in money and time to have it done and the difficulty of finding a practitioner (they are still relatively few at this

85 The gentlest, most effective pain therapy ever. *Second Opinion.* 2003;13(7):2.

time). The therapy is apparently so relaxing for the patient that many patients get drowsy on the table, and might get a bit lightheaded for just a moment when they stand. Those are my kind of risks. If they're yours, as well, you might want to track down a practitioner as soon as possible.

You can do so at bowentherapytechnique.com. Just click on "Practitioners" in the left margin, and then click on your state, province, or country when the new page comes up.

Pain Neutralization Technique

Another light-touch manipulation technique is Pain Neutralization Technique (PNT).[86] The developer of this technique is Stephen Kaufman, DC, of Denver, Colorado. His technique is so efficacious that it often relieves patients of even severe chronic pain in as little as 20 seconds.

That sounds far too good to be true, but there is a good deal of eyewitness testimony regarding the efficacy of the procedure. At the 2007 meeting of the American College for Advancement in Medicine (ACAM) in Phoenix, Dr. Kaufman put his technique on display. He treated a number of the physicians there, and subsequently obtained testimonials from most of those treated. A doctor who had suffered pain resulting from hernia surgery experienced complete resolution virtually immediately: "It took him 15-30 seconds to absolutely eradicate it."

"Dr. Kenneth A. Wolkoff, MD (from Park City, Utah) wrote: 'I had an amazing, instantaneous release of infraspinatus trigger points that have never been without pain. I've had 10 neck injuries, 40 years of neck pain and degenerated C5-6 disc. Treatment has resulted in immediate relaxation.'

"But these weren't the only cases. I saw about 40 consecutive cases of chronic pain completely resolved right in front of my eyes. The technique even resolved a few organ dysfunctions, which I thought would be impossible."[87]

Here's how an eye-witness describes the technique:

"While there are a number of techniques, the simplest one to describe involves only a specific stimulation of the muscle's trigger point. When Dr. Kaufman stimulates a muscle in a specific manner, the nervous system will automatically respond by relaxing that muscle. For instance, if you have a trigger area in your back, Dr. Kaufman identifies the muscle. He then stimulates one of a few different reflexes to that muscle. There are nerve receptors in your tendons that automatically perceive the stimulus. They reflex into your spinal cord to instantly cause the muscle to relax. This instantly breaks the circuit of painful contraction.

"If this doesn't work, Dr. Kaufman turns to an opposing muscle and uses a variety of simple reflexes on it. That makes your nervous system think that the opposing muscle is

---

86   Rowen R. Chronic pain relief in just 20 seconds. *Second Opinion.* 2008;18(6).
87   Ibid.

contracting. So, the corresponding reflex will be to instantly relax the affected muscle to allow the opposing action. Dr. Kaufman will press on the painful area or trigger point with one hand. With his other, he simultaneously applies a stimulus to the tendon of that muscle, or opposing muscles until you say 'the painful point doesn't hurt anymore.' That tells him he has found the source of the abnormal painful reflex. He simply stimulates that reflex for about 20 seconds."

Dr. Jonathan Wright confirms the incredible results from this therapy, saying results can be had in a slightly longer time period (10 minutes).[88] One of the *surgeons* in his Tahoma Clinic was so impressed with the results that he took Dr. Kaufman's course and now uses the technique extensively.

Dr. Kaufman is teaching his technique by DVD sets, available at his Web site. If your local health professional is interested in learning Bowen therapy, he or she can go to http://painneutralization.com/ and order the appropriate DVDs there. The cost at this writing ranges from $1,297 to $4,882, depending on the level of instruction desired. Alternately, your health professional could order the DVDs for you, as this is a technique that lay people could learn. Or you can call Dr. Kaufman's office for the name of a practitioner near you. The response is not terribly fast, but you should be able to get the name of a nearby practitioner this way.

* * *

These therapies and techniques that make use of very light touch to eliminate major sources of pain and set right major bodily systems are simply amazing. Aside from homeopathy, it's hard to identify a field of medicine in which so much is accomplished with so little. Obviously, with such light forces brought to bear, their potential for harm is virtually nil. As a result, their reward/risk ratio is extremely high – almost absurdly so given the high-risk environment in which most of modern medicine is conducted.

---

88   Wright JE. Eliminate pain and bring lasting relief for chronic pain sufferers in as little as ten minutes flat. *Nutrition & Healing*. wrightnewsletter.com/2013/05/22/eliminate-chronic-pain-in-minutes. Accessed September 2, 2013.

Massage Therapy

Many things in this world wear down more slowly when they're moderately used and properly maintained than when they're left idle (or extensively used or used without maintenance, for that matter). That truism is not applicable to fine china or books, but it's true of car engines and factories, for example. We've all seen cars that have been left on blocks in someone's yard for many years or factories that have been long idled. They're completely inoperable, and they take a good deal of restoration before they're useable again.

The human body is similar in this regard. It's made for use, and it must be used to remain usable. Athletes who rigorously use and condition their bodies are typically *better* able to use them than couch potatoes, not worse. We all know this, but it's an important concept.

Sometimes, though, whether because we've been on the couch too long, an injury has sidelined us, or extraordinary stress causes us to sit and stew for an extended period, we let our bodies be inactive for a long time. When that happens, we're like the car on blocks in the yard. We need some restorative work. This is where massage therapy can be invaluable. It's not the only use for massage, by a long shot, but it's a very good one.

The problem is that people who have been inactive for a long time are often either overweight or older, or both. They therefore face a problem because the forces on their joints are greater and their joints are weaker than a young, in-shape person. This is when many joint injuries occur. It's why, if you find yourself in this situation, you must get back into shape gently. People who grew up in the no-pain, no-gain school of discipline have difficulty with this. They get to the end of a long period of inactivity, get disgusted with themselves, and go out and run three miles and then lift heavy weights. The next day they're too sore to move, and the day after that they're unable to do anything without excruciating pain. As hard as it is on the muscles, it's worse on the joints. It causes injuries that might not completely heal.

When you find yourself in a state of weakness due to prolonged inactivity, you need to get things moving again *gently*. You can do this on your own if you know what you're doing or you know how to move carefully and assess what's happening as you're doing it. But if your inactivity was caused by injury or you're prone to injury because of some localized or general tissue weakness, massage can be a wonderful tool for getting things going again.

A good massage therapist can cause long-disused muscles to relax and lengthen, thus reducing stress on joints. They can induce this same effect on muscles tightened by stress. They can also move limbs without the stress of weight bearing, thus lubricating the joints and improving the range and freedom of movement. In short, they can prepare the body for physical activity, and even induce some gentle, restorative, and beneficial activity.

The human lymph system is a marvelous thing. It's a parallel circulatory system to the cardiovascular system, but it's different in composition and function. Lymph is a clear-to-white liquid that derives from interstitial fluid in the body. Interstitial fluid is literally fluid in the interstices – spaces – between the cells. It constantly takes waste material from the cells and delivers nutrition to them as it interacts with blood from capillaries. But it also interacts with lymph vessels, and carries bacteria from the cells to the lymph nodes, where it is destroyed.

Lymph is a major part of the body's immune system, and it circulates through the body much as blood does. Unlike blood, however, it does not circulate in a closed system (it rather reacts constantly with blood and lymph vessels and openly surrounds all tissue cells in the body) and it does not have a pump such as the heart. Since it does not have a pump to move it regardless of circumstance, it depends for its circulation on the expansion and contraction of muscles within the body. In short, physical activity moves the lymph. When you're not in motion, your lymph is not in motion (that's a bit of an oversimplification, but the concept is accurate).

The advantages of therapeutic massage to an injured or immobilized person can therefore hardly be exaggerated. What the body can't do because of immobility, a massage can in large measure accomplish. Both blood and lymph circulation can be improved greatly, providing greater nutrient and oxygen flow to an injury, while also providing greater white blood cell flow to the injury and taking away waste and infection from the site. These are all highly therapeutic effects, all the more so when the patient's movements are greatly restricted.

Massage also causes muscles to relax. This can be a critical effect for many injuries and conditions. It's why massage is so helpful a counter to stress. Stress can cause many muscles (especially in the neck and shoulders) to tighten to the point where they're almost as hard as a body-builder's bicep. This is one thing if you're trying to impress the judges; it's entirely another when you can't unflex the muscle. It causes exhaustion, which in turn lowers the body's resistance to disease and injury.

By causing the affected muscles to relax, these adverse effects are prevented. Stress on joints is also relieved as the muscles lengthen and stop pulling on their attachment points at the joints. This greatly increases a joint's ability to withstand the forces of life it encounters as it obeys the commands the brain issues. A relaxed knee can much better withstand a surprise step off the curb than a knee stretched taut by tense and exhausted muscles. Likewise, an already-injured knee can recuperate much faster when it is not being constantly subjected to intense tension from stress-contracted muscles. And since tendons connect muscles to bone, relaxed muscles greatly reduce the incidence of tendon injuries.

If you have a problem with chiropractic or osteopathic adjustments and the problem lasts for any length of time, it could be because your muscles are pulling the joint out of adjustment by contracting because of stress or pain. To deal with this problem, you might try getting a massage first. Tell the massage therapist what the chiropractor or osteopathic physician will be doing and what the problem has been. Massaging the muscles involved can often relax them enough to cause them to stop applying counterproductive pressure to the joints being adjusted. This will give the body more time to heal the joint, and over time could mean the difference between success and failure.

The intent of the services provided by people who provide massage to other people runs the gamut from pleasure to very serious therapy. Some services, of course, are geared strictly to stress relief and relaxation, and some to highly therapeutic effects. As beneficial as stress relief and relaxation are, if you're in pain, you probably need the next level of massage. For that, you need a massage therapist. Fortunately, this is a popular profession, and many talented people have flooded into the field. You can go to the Web site for the American Massage Therapy Association at amtamassage.org and enter your hometown or zip code. All local massage therapists who are members of this organization will be listed. Their specialties will also be listed, which will give you a good idea of the breadth and depth of skill, training, and technique available. According to the AMTA, these are the four most common types of massage available:

- Swedish: The most common type of massage, to relax and energize you.

- Deep tissue: For muscle damage from an injury, such as whiplash or back strain.

- Sports: To help prevent athletic injury, keep the body flexible and help recovery.

- Chair: Massage of the upper body, while fully clothed and seated in a special portable chair.

But many other, more specialized types of massage are common. A few of these, just to indicate the richness of the field, include:

- Cancer/oncology massage – individualized massage to improve oncology patients' relaxation, sleep, and immune function, while relieving anxiety and lessening pain, fatigue, and nausea.

- Lymphatic drainage – massage geared to moving lymph through its proper circulation to enhance lymph regeneration, reduce edema, and improve the immune system.

- Myofascial release – massage to treat the myofascia (connective tissue covering the muscles) to relieve strong pressures that cause pain throughout the body.

- Orthopedic massage – assessment, manipulation, and movement of soft tissues to resolve pain and dysfunction.

- Trigger point therapy – the treatment of small knots that develop in muscles when they are injured or overworked.

- Movement education – studying the patient's movement idiosyncrasies and training them to increase and improve their normal range of movement.

Alternatively, and perhaps optimally if you don't have good recommendations from people you know and trust, many chiropractors hire massage therapists to work in their offices. This gives you one more level of quality control, as the chiropractor will likely make sure he or she hires a good therapist. Services often run from $50 to $100 per hour, with half-hour appointments available, cheaper, and a good alternative.

If you have enough strength to do bodyweight exercises (such as pushups, stomach crunches, leg lifts, etc.), one alternative you might look into is the use of a foam roller. These are typically moderately hard to hard foam cylindrical rollers about six inches in diameter. Some are smooth and some are textured. The basic technique is to place the roller on the floor, suspend yourself over the roller with the tight muscle – the one you wish to relax – positioned on top of the roller, rest some or all of your body weight on the roller, and roll back and forth to massage the affected area. There are important considerations to make sure you don't hurt another part of your body, but most rollers have instruction manuals regarding correct technique included with the product. You can find both products and techniques listed prolifically on the Internet, or you can pick up a roller at your local sports store. Mine was a pretty basic model at Sports Authority, and was $45.

Physical Therapists, Athletic Trainers, and Exercise Physiologists

I'll discuss in this single section three disciplines that are distinct, but often have a good deal of overlap. They are included in this section because, though they tend to focus on rehabilitative exercises, they also do some limited massage and manipulation. Further, their exercise training is often hands-on, as necessary and appropriate.

Physical therapists (PTs) and exercise physiologists (EPs) are typically tied in fairly securely with the conventional medical establishment, as they work with a diagnosis provided by a doctor. Though they might find additional information as they work with the patient, their starting point and primary focus is the diagnosis they receive.

EPs typically require a higher level of education than do PTs, depending on state regulations, and they often have access to more exercise and lab equipment. Basically, both disciplines are involved with rehabilitative exercise to bring ill or injured people back up to a normal level of operation. Once they are told by a physician what the problem is, they work with the patient to do rehabilitative exercises appropriate for the patient's condition. Like osteopathic physicians and chiropractors, EPs and PTs benefit from an explosion in understanding of human physiology over the past two or three decades. As a result, their exercises and techniques are typically highly efficacious. And because they are closely associated with doctors, if you find a good doctor, you will usually be referred to a good EP or PT.

Your standard of care is more likely to pertain to the individual involved and their professionalism and degree of diligence and understanding than on the designation they work under (PT or EP). Either is capable of bringing a great deal of value to your recuperation efforts. That said, an EP has typically gone through more training than a PT.

If you're well acquainted with exercise basics and pay close attention to the "If it hurts, don't do that" rule, there are a number of illustrated therapeutic exercises listed on Web sites, as mentioned in the bulleted suggestion portion of the section on exercise. It's likely you can do yourself a lot of good, even if you can't for some reason go to an exercise physiologist or a physical therapist. However, an EP/PT can usually tailor the exercises you should do to your injury more specifically, and they can give you feedback on how you are doing the exercises, which will help you avoid injuring yourself further by doing them incorrectly.

The third discipline mentioned in this section, athletic trainer, is quite an interesting one – and one well worth your time to look into. It may be the ultimate medical resource. America's love affair with sports of all stripes has occasioned much of the increase in knowledge of the body and how it works. The rise of extreme sports; the popularity of contact sports such as football, rugby, and hockey; and the high levels of competition that require optimum performance and rapid recovery from injury have all demanded huge increases in knowledge and technology. Athletic trainers are often on the front lines of this process, and the demands placed on them are commensurate with serious and frequent injuries, as well as efficacious and diverse recuperative techniques.

Many amateur teams do not have the luxury of a team doctor, at least not one who can always be on the field with the team, so they employ athletic trainers (and many teams with full-time doctors also employ ATs). These professionals are trained in baccalaureate level college programs that require specific courses of study and provide a degree in athletic training. The consequence is a degreed, certified professional who obtains intense training in an environment where injuries happen often, are frequently significant, and are occasionally quite serious. It's no place for the weak of mind or stomach. And it produces some very serious-minded, capable, and broadly educated individuals.

The upshot of all this for you is that many of these professionals also see non-athletes or non-team-associated athletes as a separate aspect of their practice. Unlike EPs or PTs, ATs often provide their own diagnoses. This can save you time and money, and get you on the road to recuperation sooner. Further, in their capacity as team trainers, these individuals often have vast networks of other health professionals they can call on – and they can call on them at odd hours, as athletic teams often play at night or on weekends.

A friend of mine, who is an AT and has helped me numerous times with my back problem, was once an AT for Northwestern University in Chicago. At that time, he had a well-established network of 64 health professionals that he could call on for treatment related to his diagnosis, or for further and more detailed diagnosis. He referred me to the chiropractor and the osteopathic physician I now see. To see him in his non-team-related capacity cost a small fraction of what it would cost to see a physician in an office setting (actually, he didn't charge me at all, but would have charged only $50 had he not been a close friend), and access to supportive help was extensive, if it was needed.

This same friend recently taught a series of classes called range of motion (ROM) training, which I attended. From a functional standpoint, physiologically, this was the most productive thing I've done in decades. It entailed a series of exercises that gently but firmly involved muscles and joints that are typically left to atrophy in normal adult life.

When we are young, we engage in many activities that keep our entire range of muscles and connective tissues in shape. Whether it's wrestling, team sports, ballet, or any of myriad other activities, we are stretched, twisted, and otherwise contorted into total functional condition. As we age, our lives tend to gravitate toward straight forward or straight up and down activity. We sit, we stand, we walk, we jog, we bicycle, we swim, but we seldom flex or twist to the left or the right. This causes us to become very fragile and easily hurt if we deviate with any force from these accustomed axes of movement. And perhaps more importantly from the standpoint of pain, we are not able to adequately recover from injury if we do not train the oblique muscles that support our injured joints.

ROM training is designed to do precisely such training of oblique muscles, even as it increases flexibility. It also puts mild stress on the joints in oblique directions, which strengthens them against injury or obesity-related stress.[89] One man in my class who had undergone double knee replacement surgery found the exercises so beneficial that he give up his physical therapy entirely. This is not necessarily recommended, but is one indication of how helpful the exercises can be. If you're able to work with a good AT, be sure to ask them about ROM training and how you can take advantage of it.

ATs benefit from the environment in which they work. Sports medicine in general tends to have less political and medical-industrial baggage than many other forms of medicine. It is far from free of it, but a pragmatic "whatever works" approach reigns supreme in sports (or at least tries to). For this reason, professional athletes are often early adopters of, and provide many early-stage testimonials for, new, cutting-edge therapies. This has been apparent in some of the write-ups in this report. Thus, athletes and the health professionals who attend them tend to be more open to new and not-yet-exhaustively-proven therapies. ATs are often prime beneficiaries of this results-oriented mindset.

Without the peer pressure that arises from a medical doctor's 11 to 18 years of specialized

---

89   Earlier in this report, I extolled the virtues of bicycling precisely because it limited the range of motion that was possible. Compared to this information on ROM training, that recommendation might be confusing. It's not meant to be. Each exercise has its place, and limited range of motion exercise can be done as you build up to ROM training after an injury, or concurrently with ROM training. I do the latter, using stationary bicycle training for its cardio-vascular and leg-strengthening benefits, at the same time doing ROM training for the benefits it provides. A toolkit should have many tools for various purposes and needs, and bicycling is just as valuable as ROM training, but needs to be balanced in its use.

education, ATs are less bound to pursue only conventional treatments. This varies from individual to individual, of course, but many are open to whatever can be demonstrated to restore health quickly and thoroughly. Such a person can be a very good individual to know, as he or she will probably be far more intensively immersed in the treatment of injuries than you might be, and will be able to give you rehabilitative exercises for your injury without the diagnosis of a doctor. An AT will also know people in your area who can provide the best possible treatment for your injury if more extensive care is required, and will know how those people have treated patients in the past. If you can make the acquaintance of an AT, you will have an excellent and inexpensive option when you hurt yourself and need help quickly.

Finding an AT can be a bit of a challenge. The National Athletic Trainers Association maintains a Web site at nata.org, but does not provide a membership list or list of practitioners by location. Your local yellow pages will not likely have a listing for them, either. You can start by contacting your local high school or college football coach and asking them for contact information for their athletic trainer, if they have one. Or you can call a sports doctor and ask if he or she knows of a good athletic trainer in the area. Other than that, the grapevine is often the best option. If you don't have a health grapevine, you might want to consider starting one. It can be a priceless resource for identifying good local health practitioners and telling others about them. All it takes is a few friends and acquaintances, or a few online contacts, who like to talk about their experiences with health practitioners and therapies.

Part 4

Miscellaneous Helpful Therapies

As helpful as are the broad categories of treatment that we have dealt with thus far, there are many excellent therapies that do not easily fit into them. I'll mention a few of the more important ones here in the interest of covering as many options as possible.

Chapter 15

Honey

Given that honey tastes so good, it's often surprising to find that it has such strong therapeutic use. Many bee products have health uses, from propolis to royal jelly. But plain old honey is surprising in its antibacterial properties. One reason for this is that it contains hydrogen peroxide, and we've discussed the strongly antibacterial properties of that substance earlier.

Recently, however, it's been found that honey varies quite a bit in its antibacterial and healing qualities, and that the honey that comes from the manuka tree in New Zealand has the strongest antibacterial properties.[90] Several companies market this honey now, and they do so primarily for its therapeutic uses, not for dietary use. It has proved to be so effective in healing skin damage from aging and the sun that it's also being added to many skin care products.

That said, most honeys have antibacterial properties, and can be used to relieve pain and heal wounds quickly. Get the manuka honey if you can, but don't hesitate to use whatever is at hand. Diabetic ulcers respond especially well to honey. Cuts, abrasions, burns, open sores, and other skin wounds are also well served by smearing honey over the wound and then bandaging it to keep dirt and debris out but allow air in. People who have had their diabetic ulcers so treated report that the pain subsides almost immediately.

An old folk remedy is also said to be therapeutic for arthritis. Mix two teaspoons of honey with two teaspoons of cider vinegar in one cup of warm water. Drink this mixture three times a day. It might take a few weeks to see results, but the combination is widely reported to be helpful.

---

90   Williams D. Get a honey of a complexion. *Alternatives*. 2008;12(15):118.

Chapter 16

Drop Therapy

Several years ago, my wife developed severe pain in the center of her chest. That was quite alarming, of course, and we had two different cardiologists check her out. Both said she was fine; nothing was wrong. The pain continued. It was an extremely difficult and frustrating time.

I was publishing Dr. David Williams' newsletter *Alternatives* at the time, and an article came to my attention suggesting that some chest pain that seems heart-related might in fact be a hiatal hernia. This happens when part of the stomach pushes up through the diaphragm at the point where the esophagus passes through it on its way from the mouth to the stomach. That point is called the hiatus. If the stomach herniates and pushes up through the diaphragm into the chest cavity, it can be quite painful. In many cases, it can mimic heart pain.

The solution for this is to drink a glass of warm or room temperature water (12 ounces or more) first thing when you get up in the morning. Then, says, Dr. Williams, "While standing, bring your arms straight out from your sides and bend your elbows so your hands are touching your chest. Then stand up on your toes as high as possible and drop. You should get a pretty good jolt. Drop down 10 times in a row. Then raise your arms up and pant short quick breaths for about 15 seconds. That's it."[91]

The warm water causes the stomach to relax and acts as a weight to make the stomach heavy. Spreading the arms opens up the diaphragm and the hiatus, as well. Dropping down sharply causes the water to pull the stomach down through the hiatus. And the rapid breathing causes the hiatus to close up again. Do this every day, not just until the hernia heals (and it takes a few weeks to heal – some residual pain continues for a while, though it will be obvious that the problem has been largely solved).

You can see from this procedure the logic employed in medicine that works. This is simple physics applied to biology. The reason it works is straightforward, simple, and efficacious. Many conditions and injuries do not have such a simple solution, but the laws of nature apply. If patient welfare is put ahead of process, profit, and preconceived notions, it's amazing what can be accomplished.

This worked like a charm for my wife. It took her a few weeks to get back to normal, but the severe pain resolved instantly. Our opinion of hidebound, unimaginative, peer-pressured doctors, especially those of the cardiological persuasion, sunk like a water-weighted stomach. But our appreciation for simple, straightforward medicine was greatly increased.

---

91 Williams D. Get rid of heartburn for good. Special health tip exclusively for EasyRenew Members. November 2009.

Chapter 17

Static Electricity for Arthritis

Another famous low-cost solution is to use a statically charged scrap of PVC pipe to relieve arthritis pain. Dr. David Williams contends that every cell in the body has both a positive and a negative charge. When an imbalance occurs, malfunction and some degree of disease is the consequence. Apparently it works the other way around, as well – malfunction can cause an electrical imbalance – because with inflammation, a positive electrical charge results.

To balance it, you can create a negative charge with the aforesaid PVC pipe. In my case, Home Depot had a two-foot section of ½" (internal diameter) pipe for 99¢. It worked perfectly. Just rub it briskly with a piece of fuzzy material from a craft store (that's all the description Dr. Williams provides; I was able to use a polyester material that looks similar to terrycloth; I suspect any polyester material will do), which will build up a static electrical charge. You can tell the PVC is charged by moving it over your arm; the hair will stand up as you do so. Then move the charged pipe slowly back and forth over the affected area about a half-inch away from the skin.

After moving the pipe over the skin three or four times, or after touching the skin with it (which discharges it), recharge the pipe with the fuzzy material (or polyester cloth) and pass it over the area again. Do this until the pain subsides. Most people experience relief in about five to seven minutes.[92] It didn't take that long for me, but it was surprisingly effective. The relief is not permanent, but it offers a very nice break from the pain.

---

92   Williams D. 25 solutions under $25. 25th Anniversary Editorial Insert. July 2010.

Chapter 18

Vitamin D for Back Pain

Earlier in this report, I expounded on a therapy developed by Dr. Frank Shallenberger called prolozone®. This therapy has been so spectacular in its results that he measures failure in astoundingly small numbers: "Out of hundreds, maybe thousands, of cases, there have been a handful in which the treatment did not work at all."[93] Even with such amazing success, these failures bothered him quite a bit. But he thinks he might have discovered a reason why some cases do not respond to prolozone.

His discovery came through an article in the *Journal of the American Board of Family Medicine*.[94] Six chronic severe back-pain sufferers were featured in the article. Each had experienced long-term suffering without any success from surgery or other interventions. Every single one of them responded positively to supplemental vitamin D. Some were completely healed. The responses were amazing. The article author noted that "the patients in this study who responded best used between 4,000 and 5,000 IU of vitamin D3/day."[95]

Interestingly, Dr. Shallenberger also noted that a fibromyalgia patient he had treated experienced similar results with vitamin D supplementation. She was the most vitamin D-deficient patient he had ever encountered, and he had to give her an extremely high level of daily supplementation (eventually 20,000 IU/day) to get her over 80 ng/ml, which is slightly above the minimum level he considers healthy (70 ng/ml). When she reached 80 ng/ml, her fibromyalgia symptoms virtually disappeared.[96]

If you have a chronic pain problem that resists all efforts to resolve it, find a doctor who will work with you to check and, if necessary, raise your vitamin D levels. If your level is below 70 ng/ml (not nmol/l, which is also used, but is a different measurement), raising your level of D might produce startlingly positive results. Try to spend a little time in indirect sunlight each day, as well. Twenty to thirty minutes is usually enough. The natural vitamin D your body makes when exposed to sunlight is even better than supplementation, and you can't overdose on it.

---

93   Shallenberger F. Chronic low back pain? It might be a vitamin deficiency. *Real Cures.* 2010;9(2);1.
94   Schwalfenberg G. Improvement of chronic back pain or failed back surgery with vitamin D repletion: a case series. *J Am Board Fam Med.* 2009;22:69-74. doi:10.3122/jabfm.2009.01.080026.
95   Ibid.
96   Chronic low back pain? 2.

Chapter 19

TMJ Therapy

In earlier chapters, we looked at how important oxygen is for healing. We haven't really discussed how important it is for functioning properly, and how the lack of oxygen can cause some of the very problems that might have caused you to buy this report in the first place. Almost everyone knows how important oxygen is to human health and functioning. But it turns out that many of us don't get what we need because of obstructions to our breathing. And many of those who have this condition don't even know it. Perhaps their tongue is excessively large for their mouth, their jaw is misaligned, or the muscles governing their epiglottis (the small flap at the base of the tongue that prevents food and drink from going down the trachea when swallowing) are fatigued or too weak. They can breathe, but they can't get all the oxygen their bodies need for normal – much less optimal – functioning.

A dentist in Washington state named Farrand Robson has been researching this condition and the problems that result from it. These include pain in the face, ear region, head, neck, shoulders, and back, as well as such things as fibromyalgia, sleep problems, and on-edge feelings or mental fog. It's amazing that such a host of issues could have a common cause. Systemic shortage of oxygen, however, can manifest in a large number of ways – many of them quite serious. To simply adjust the physiology of the jaw as a remedy to this problem is an amazingly logical, simple, and brilliant idea.

Dr. Robson has done precisely this. He has developed a system of treating breathing obstructions that frequently gives his patients immediate relief from such things as sleep apnea, shortness of breath, the kinds of pain mentioned above, and a surprising number of other issues. One of his patients tells his story at http://fibrofriends.typepad.com/fibro_friends/oral_systemic_balance/. The patient discusses the cost of this procedure, which is substantial, and provides a couple of pictures of the devices Dr. Robson made for him.

I hesitated to write about this therapy because it is still in its early days. Price is high and availability is low – there are apparently 30 to 40 practitioners throughout the country at this point, but you have to contact Dr. Robson's office to find one near you, and you might have to leave a message and wait and wait – literally months, as this goes to press, but they say they're working to reduce the time it takes to return calls, and hopefully that will have happened by the time you read this.

If you mention my name and this book, you might get a return call faster. And I must say it may be worth the wait, considering the remarkable results people report from this therapy. Dr.

Robson appears to be emphasizing control and quality over availability – which has merits as a strategy, but can be frustrating if you need the treatment.

You can go to oralsystembiology.com, click on the "Contact Us" button, and fill in your information to request the name of a practitioner near you, or you can call his office at 800-977-1945. You can also do an Internet search for "oral systemic balance," which is the name of his system, along with the name of your state or a neighboring one to see if any nearby practitioner has an individual Web site. My searches along those lines were disappointing – though I found a few throughout the nation – so don't be surprised if there's not yet much to find.

In the end, I decided to feature the therapy because it seems to have almost astounding breadth and depth of application. Dr. Rowen was instantly helped by the installation of a device by Dr. Robson. He wrote about a few cases where similar results were obtained by acquaintances, friends, or patients of his. His friend Ron had an extraordinary outcome:

Ron suffered from severe sleep apnea and couldn't breathe while sleeping without the help of a machine. But Dr. Robson fixed his problem with one treatment. Ron now sleeps like a baby without any help from a machine.

What did Dr. Robson do that was so miraculous? He simply put a specially made splint into Ron's mouth and, presto, Ron was breathing without help.

Ron says, "Immediately, when Dr. Robson put the splint in my mouth, I felt a release in my throat. A wave of relaxation engulfed my body. Instantly, breathing took no effort. Living in the fog of breathlessness for years, I mistook even daytime breathing effort for 'normal' and now realize that I was struggling for air even while awake. At 53, I have been reborn thanks to Dr. Robson's work!"[97]

Dr. Rowen chronicles several other miraculous outcomes in patients suffering from conditions as diverse as sleep apnea, fibromyalgia, irritable bowel syndrome, acid reflux, and neck and back pain.

The patient who wrote at the fibrofriends site listed above also had instant and highly substantive (though not comprehensive, as he notes) results. As Dr. Robson writes in the *Townsend Letter*, "Remarkable benefit for many millions of people is possible if the origin of TMJ disorders is demonstrated and then linked to the host of these somatic pain syndromes."[98] A number of remarks and observations by physicians, health professionals, and patients would seem to confirm the validity of this very ambitious statement.

97   Rowen R. New discovery relieves sleep apnea – and back pain – instantly! *Second Opinion*. 2004;14(2).
98   Robson FC. Unmasking the imposter: effective, predictable treatment for symptom sets known as TMJ, FM, and more. *Townsend Letter for Doctors and Patients*. 2005;264:90-94.

Chapter 20

Frequency Specific Modulation Therapy

FSM therapy will sound new to many readers, but is actually an old technology. It was pioneered and used in the first half of the 20th century, but was driven from the repertoire of practicing doctors by the medical cartel behind the efforts of AMA president Morris Fishbein, M.D. Anything at that time that was not reproducible, such as drugs or surgery, was purged from the list of permissible therapies.[99]

In the 1990s, however, FSM was not only resurrected, but was made even more effective than it was earlier in the century. Carolyn McMakin, D.C., discovered a list of frequencies that had been used with the original technology and had a new, more effective machine made. Dr. McMakin remains active in both using this technology and training others to use it.

FSM consists of a small machine that generates very small electrical currents, similar to, but using much smaller current than, a TENS unit. TENS, you may know, stands for transcutaneous electrical nerve stimulation, and is a therapy intended to stimulate nerves and block pain signals. In contrast, according to Nenah Sylver, Ph.D.,

"Frequency Specific Microcurrent (FSM) treats nerve, muscle, and fascia pain by using a wider range of frequencies (from 3 hertz to 970 hertz) to favorably alter tissue and restore health, using minute amounts of micro-amperage current. A TENS unit has an output of up to 100 milliamps, which can overwhelm the body with current that is easily felt. In contrast, the output of FSM is in microamps (millionths of an amp), which is not readily perceived by the body even though its effects are. (An ampere is a measure of the movement of electrons or current.) Significantly, the output of FSM imitates the output produced naturally by the body within each cell. The amount of FSM current is not strong enough to stimulate sensory nerves, so the treatment usually cannot be felt and is painless, as well as safe, non-invasive, and effective."[100]

Thus, a TENS unit decreases cell energy while FSM increases it. Its mechanism of action is similar to a Rife machine, if you're familiar with that technology, except that the Rife machine uses electromagnetic radiation in the radio frequency range, and an FSM machine uses electrical impulses. The similarity between the two technologies arises in that both machines vary the frequency of their output in order to deal with different injuries, conditions, or infections. The

---

99   Rowen R. Forgotten pain cure – once outlawed by the FDA – makes a remarkable comeback. *Second Opinion.* 2005;15(10):1.
100 Sylver N. Healing with electromedicine and sound therapies, part two. *Townsend Letter.* April 2008.

theory behind this variation is that every infectious agent has a resonant frequency that can destroy it. To understand this, consider the highly clichéd example of the soprano and the crystal wine glass. At a certain frequency, she can hit a note that causes the glass to shatter because the crystalline structure of the glass begins to wildly vibrate at that precise frequency. The brittle nature of crystal doesn't let it flex – so it shatters.

Many microscopic life forms can also be destroyed in this way, even though they're more flexible than crystal. Viruses and bacteria are of particular interest since they are such frequent disease organisms, and they can typically be destroyed at resonant frequencies that leave human cells unfazed. But human cells also have frequencies that can impart energy to them and enhance their function. FSM therefore sometimes uses two circuits that are keyed to two frequencies – one to enhance the health of the body part at issue and the second to battle the infection that is involved.[101]

As with all electrical connections, a circuit must be completed. Thus, the machine has two contacts, one positive and one negative. These contacts are placed on the body at the beginning and ending point of the intended path of the microcurrent. The current is so small that in most cases it can't even be felt, but it passes directly through the body, destroying pathogens and/or stimulating cells in its path.

Terrell Owens, wide receiver for the Philadelphia Eagles, suffered a serious ankle injury on December 19, 2004, and was sidelined as a result. But he underwent immediate and ongoing FSM therapy, and healed with almost surreal speed as a result. (FSM is most helpful if you can begin it within four hours of a surgery or injury.)

By the time of the Super Bowl on February 6, 2005, Owens was not only able to play, but had nine receptions for 122 yards – a 13.6 yard-per-catch average. Doing this against the Super Bowl-champion New England Patriots was clearly very high-level play within less than two months of a possible career-ending injury. Owens gave FSM much of the credit for his stunning recovery.

Professional golfer Bill Glassen also experienced remarkable healing with FSM. His small plane was struck by lightning, which resulted in mental fog so serious he couldn't concentrate – even so much as to balance a checkbook. He also experienced pain throughout his body, particularly in his knees. Two knee surgeries didn't improve a thing – because the problem wasn't there. His brain and nervous system were the source of the problem, but no therapy he tried helped.

After years of suffering, he went to Dr. McMakin for FSM therapy. She treated him for five hours a day over the course of three days. "The results were so miraculous that he was able to begin playing golf again. He's been on the pro tour ever since, and finished a tournament in

---

101 Rowen R. Reverse heart disease, macular degeneration, and any chronic pain in minutes. *Second Opinion.* 2005;15(11):2.

fourth place out of 250 competitors. He was so impressed by the FSM machine that he bought a home unit."[102]

Speaking of home units, they are available, but they're not cheap. As with some of the other therapies mentioned in this report, competition has not been well established in the manufacture of these units. Since they are FDA approved, that is probably the competition killer in this case. Getting a specific device approved is not automatic, even though the therapy itself has been approved. (FSM units are considered TENS units for the purpose of regulation, though they emit a far smaller current, as we discussed earlier.)

Manufacturers are listed in the resources section. Hopefully, other FSM machine makers will enter the field as the treatment becomes more widespread. In the meantime, you can find an FSM practitioner near you by going to Dr. McMakin's site at frequencyspecific.com/practitioners. php and entering your city and state, or zip code. The practitioner in my town charges $75 for an hour of FSM treatment.

---

102 Reverse heart disease; 1.

Chapter 21

How to Get a Good Night's Sleep In Spite of Chronic Pain

Often, one of the most problematic things about suffering pain is that it robs you of sleep. It's bad enough to hurt; it's worse when you can't get enough rest. After you've tried some of the therapies in this report, one other thing you can work on is your sleeping situation – by which I mean the mattress and pillows you sleep on.

There are a multitude of opinions on this subject, and many of them are too inflexible. Clearly, individualism is a big factor in this matter. For instance, many chiropractors, D.O.s, and other back experts advise people with back pain to sleep on a firm mattress. This works for many people. Not me. Not only does it make my back hurt, it makes everything hurt.

The most comfortable night's sleep I've had in the last 30 years was when I went to a family camping weekend that was held at a Girl Scout camp in the mountains. The only bed available had a spring-and-wire base with a 2½" thick, very soft, cheap foam pad on it. I put another identical pad on top of that one, spread my sleeping bag on top of the lot, and slept like a baby.

My theory on why this worked so well is this: With no tucked-in sheet on the bed, there was no "skin tension" to keep the soft mattresses from conforming thoroughly to my body contours. The sleeping bag was a soft down one, so it also conformed very well. Thus, rather than being supported at three or four points (generally head, shoulder, hip, and leg), I was supported at just about every point of my body that lay within two or three inches of the bed surface. This felt wonderful, and I don't believe I shifted my position the whole night long. No soreness from a pressure point developed, so I didn't need to shift. Additionally, and perhaps most importantly, my back felt great the next morning. I think that the same "complete support" concept was responsible for that outcome.

If you sleep well with a firm mattress, stay with it. From what I understand, most people do well with such support, and I don't want to mess with your success. But if you toss and turn a lot at night, develop pressure points, or have pain because your injured or painful body part is not well supported while you sleep, a very soft mattress is something worth trying.

Alternatively, if your injury is on a limb, you might want to try some very soft pillows to support it while you sleep. Feather pillows are about as soft as they come, so try stacking a few in various positions that feel good to you. When you find a position that relieves the pain, chances are you've taken stress off of the injury and you'll both sleep and heal better.

The key with this concept is to customize your rest and sleep positions with mattress and/or pillow options that minimize your pain. This will take some experimentation. It helps if you have a number of pillows at hand and another person to help you adjust them. Try to find a position that doesn't hurt and in which you can sleep, and then try to support that position with pillows, as necessary.

Mattresses are a bit harder to research, though many companies are trying to make it easier. Some allow you to sleep for several weeks on their mattress without committing to keep it. Alternatively, if you visit family or friends and sleep on a mattress that agrees with you, ask them what kind it is.

To see if the soft mattress concept agrees with you, try inflating an old-fashioned camping air mattress, but inflate it only about half way. Put it on your mattress (if any of your joints or limbs touch the ground due to the low level of inflation, it helps to have them rest on a bed rather than the hard ground), and sleep on it with either a loose sheet covering it or, as I did, a soft sleeping bag. If this agrees with you, chances are you'll enjoy a soft mattress as much as I do.

I've become a big fan of latex mattresses. They're comfortable and durable (many last 30 or 40 years without discernible wear). Because the latex is heated quite a bit during the manufacturing process, the protein that causes latex allergies is changed in nature. Thus, few (if any) people have any problems with allergies to latex mattresses. And they're typically perforated so they breathe well. They're neither hot in the summer nor cold in the winter.

Latex comes in various levels of firmness. Obviously, I favor the soft ones. Even so, it's not as soft as the cheap stuff at Girl Scout camps. For that, you need to order a soft density type of foam from a company like Foam N' More at foamforyou.com/Open_Cell_Foam.htm. The good thing is that this kind of foam is truly cheap. The bad thing is that it's not durable. It'll last a few years at most. If you get great sleep for a couple of years for the price, however, that's not such a bad thing.

This kind of foam is also treated for fire retardancy, so there are chemicals in it that your skin can absorb. Almost all mattresses are now treated, but companies don't tend to customize the cheap mattresses, so it's hard, if not impossible, to get an untreated one. This is therefore a tough problem to solve without lessening the ability of the foam to conform to your body. Using two or three sheets laid on top (not tightly tucked around the sides) will help without creating too much skin tension. I'd recommend washing the sheets often to keep them from becoming sources of the chemicals themselves.

An adjustable bed is a great option if you can afford it. It will elevate your upper body and knees to just the right angle for relief, watching TV, or reading, and return the bed to horizontal when you choose. If you choose not to purchase an adjustable bed, but would like to elevate your torso and knees, you can get foam wedges to help you do so. They're much cheaper, and can be had from companies like Foam N' More at foamforyou.com/back_support_wedges. htm#Body%20Wedges.

Memory foam is a popular form of support foam these days. It largely performs as advertised, but for only a short time. It is a plastic rather than a rubber, which means it has substantially weaker cell structure than rubber-based products such as latex. It can't maintain its structural integrity for very long – a couple of years to perhaps four, depending on the quality of materials used. Mine lasted only about two or three before it began sagging and subjecting me to the hammock effect – which is not good for the back. It's rather expensive stuff, given its limited lifespan.

Most mattresses are treated with flame retardants, as required by law these days. The chemicals used to do this can be quite harmful to health, as explained very thoughtfully by Lee Carter in his video at mattresseducation.net. Some companies provide untreated mattresses if you can produce a doctor's statement that you have skin sensitivities that require you to sleep on a non-chemically treated mattress. Lee's company does this, though it does not offer the cheap foam types of mattress. His products are chemical-free, well made, and pricey. If you want the best, he's your man. If price is a factor, other options are listed in the Resources section.

Conclusion

Though pain is such a huge part of life, and there are so many kinds and intensities of it, its treatment seems to come down to just a few basics: Good nutrition, appropriate exercise, and the selective use of electromagnetic radiation, physical manipulation, and oxygen. Add to these a few essential oils, some DMSO, some honey, a good mattress, some good chairs, lots of soft pillows, and a few other key items, and you'll be ready for a host of possibilities. When guided by clear, serious, and informed thinking, it's a potent toolkit with extremely wide and deep application. Though the "cut, burn, and poison" (surgery, chemotherapy, and drugs) school of conventional medicine has a place, that place is currently *far* bigger than it ought to be.

If tomorrow America decided to elect governments at all levels that did not have the desire to totally control people, and if we instituted an honest economic system, the elements of these five therapeutic categories would rapidly fall in price and increase in availability. Economics is that powerful. The prevalence of conscientious practitioners who would compete for customer allegiance based on competence and price would also increase. It would be a much better world, but right now it's pie in the sky. It won't happen because most people just don't think that way. And without coherent citizen demand, governments have no incentive to change.

So those who do see the situation accurately must take matters into their own hands. They must invest in their own education, buying and studying materials such as this report. They must invest in their own health, eating good food and exercising thoughtfully and often. They must purchase such medical products and devices as their conditions require and their budgets allow, and use them to restore health when it is lost. They must find support networks of like-minded people, and exceptional physicians to help them when help is needed. And lastly, they must selectively tell others about these matters. After over two decades in the information business, I'm under no illusions about people's willingness to hear information that runs counter to their fundamental belief that people in control are good and are here to help us. Trying to tell them differently is almost always an exercise in tilting at windmills. But some people will listen, and they should be told.

Americans' blind faith in their leaders, together with the corruption that that uncritical faith has enabled, are about to yield their inevitable fruit – failure. And crisis has a way of challenging people's most fundamental beliefs. Perhaps when healthcare is poor and hard to come by (even more so than now), more people will listen to reason. Perhaps they will understand that the rule of law, personal responsibility, and private property are the only bases on which to establish institutions that work. I hope so. I'm not holding my breath, but I hope so.

In the meantime, I hope this report helps you to relieve your pain and restore your health. That is its purpose, and your success will be the measure of mine. Keep at it, and learn from both your pain and the therapies you use to relieve it. Whole new realms of knowledge, activity, accomplishment, and meaning will open up as you do so.

Section 3

Resources

Many of these resources have only an Internet presence (they do not publicize a physical address or a phone number). If you don't have a computer or an Internet connection, you can look these sources up on a computer at the library or have a friend or family member help you on their computer.

Aquaponics

- Backyard Aquaponics: backyardaquaponics.com/

- Friendly Aquaponics: friendlyaquaponics.com/

- Portable Farms: http://portablefarms.com/

Backyard Gardening

- The astounding power of mulch (superb free video): backtoedenfilm.com/

- The urban homestead – what can be done in a small city yard (three tons per year of organic produce from a 1/10-acre garden): http://urbanhomestead.org/

Books Describing Diets Modeled on Healthy Populations

- *The Okinawa Program: How the World's Longest-Lived People Achieve Everlasting Health – And How You Can Too*, by Bradley J. Willcox and Makoto Suzuki

- *The MediterrAsian Way: A Cookbook and Guide to Health, Weight Loss, and Longevity, Combining the Best Features of Mediterranean and Asian Diets*, by Trudy Thelander and Ric Watson

- *The Mediterranean Prescription: Meal Plans and Recipes to Help You Stay Slim and Healthy for the Rest of Your Life,* Hardcover, by Angelo Acquista with Laurie Anne Vandermolen

- These and many others on the same subjects available at amazon.com

Environmental Medicine – For information on medical professionals who diagnose and treat medical issues stemming from environmental sources, including toxins, molds, allergens, etc.

- The American Academy of Environmental Medicine
  6505 E. Central Avenue, #296
  Wichita, KS 67206
  Tel: 316-684-5500
  http://aaemonline.org/

- The American Board of Environmental Medicine
  65 Wehrle Drive, Buffalo, NY 14225
  Tel: 716.833.2213
  Fax: 716.833.2244
  americanboardofenvironmentalmedicine.org/certification.htm

FSM Machines

- Forrest Health
  408-354-4262
  forresthealth.com/inspirstar-microcurrent-stimulator-programmed.html

- Senergy Medical Group
  9901 Valley Ranch Parkway East, Suite 1009
  Irving, TX 75063
  972-580-0545
  senergy.us/biomodulator-devices.html

Mattresses and Foam Products

- Dreamfoam Bedding
  Available only on Amazon.com
  chuck@dreamfoam.com

- Foam Factory
  586-627-3626
  carlo@foambymail.com
  foambymail.com
  (Decent, inexpensive products; customer service not superb)

- Foam N' More Inc.
  1177 W. Maple Rd.
  Clawson, MI 48017
  866-212-6552
  http://foamforyou.com/
  (Treated products only.)

- Sleep Essentials, Inc.
  3542 Orange Avenue
  Roanoke, VA 24012
  540-397-2337
  Lee@sleepessentials.com
  http://perfectlatexmattress.com

Multivitamins, High-Quality

- Daily Advantage, formulated by Dr. David Williams
  Tel: 1-800-844-2117
  drdavidwilliams.com/daily-advantage/

- Forward Plus, formulated by Julian Whitaker, M.D.
  Tel: 1-800-804-0936
  drwhitaker.com/forward-plus/

- Healthy Resolve, formulated by Robert Rowen, M.D.
  Tel: 800-791-3395
  advancedbionutritionals.com

- Quickstart DM, formulated by Frank Shallenberger, M.D.
  Tel: 775-884-3990
  antiagingmedicine.com/cart/product-list/quickstart-dm.html

Physicians

- Jorge D. Flechas, M.D. (fibromyalgia specialist)
  Flechas Family Practice
  #80 Doctors Drive, Suite 3
  Hendersonville, NC 28792
  828-684-3233
  ffplabnc1@live.com
  helpmythyroid.com

- Robert Rowen, M.D.
  2200 County Center Drive
  Santa Rosa, CA 95403
  707-578-7787

- Frank Shallenberger, M.D.
  The Nevada Center of Alternative & Anti-Aging Medicine
  1231 Country Club Drive
  Carson City NV 89703
  775-884-3990
  antiagingmedicine.com

- Julian Whitaker, M.D.
  Whitaker Wellness Institute
  4321 Birch St.
  Newport Beach, CA 92660
  866-944-8253
  info@whitakerwellness.com
  whitakerwellness.com